CRYSTAL
PRESCRIPTIONS

Volume 6

Crystals for Karmic Healing, Soul
Reintegration and Ancestral Clearing.
An A-Z Guide

T0095912

CRYSTAL
PRESCRIPTIONS

Volume 6

Crystals for Karmic Healing, Soul
Reintegration and Ancestral Clearing.
An A-Z Guide

Judy Hall

Author of the best-selling

The Crystal Bible series

BOOKS

Winchester, UK
Washington, USA

JOHN HUNT PUBLISHING

First published by O-Books, 2017
O-Books is an imprint of John Hunt Publishing Ltd., 3 East St., Alresford,
Hampshire SO24 9EE, UK
office@jhpbooks.com
www.johnhuntpublishing.com
www.o-books.com

For distributor details and how to order please visit the 'Ordering' section on our
website.

ISBN: 978 1 78535 455 7
978 1 78535 456 4 (ebook)

A CIP catalogue record for this book is available from the British Library.

Design: Stuart Davies

UK: Printed and bound by CPI Group (UK) Ltd, Croydon, CR0 4YY
US: Printed and bound by Thomson-Shore, 7300 West Joy Road, Dexter, MI 48130

We operate a distinctive and ethical publishing philosophy
in all areas of our business, from our global network of
authors to production and worldwide distribution.

CONTENTS

Volumes in this series:

Crystal Prescriptions

The A–Z guide to over 1,200 symptoms and their healing crystals
ISBN: 978-1-90504-740-6 (Paperback) £7.99 $15.95

Crystal Prescriptions volume 2

The A–Z guide to over 1,250 conditions and their new
generation healing crystals
ISBN: 978-1-78279-560-5 (Paperback) £8.99 $14.95

Crystal Prescriptions volume 3

Crystal solutions to electromagnetic pollution and geopathic stress.
An A–Z guide.
ISBN: 978-1-78279-791-3 (Paperback) £8.99 $14.95

Crystal Prescriptions volume 4

The A–Z guide to the chakra balancing crystals and kundalini
activation stones
ISBN: 978-1-78535-053-5 (Paperback) £10.99 $17.95

Crystal Prescriptions volume 5

Space clearing, Feng Shui and Psychic Protection.
An A-Z guide.
ISBN: 978-1-78535-457-1 (Paperback) £12.99 $19.95

Crystal Prescriptions volume 6

Crystals for ancestral clearing, soul retrieval, spirit release and karmic
healing. An A-Z guide.
ISBN: 978-1-78535-455-7 (Paperback) £13.99 $19.95

Crystal Prescriptions volume 7

The A-Z Guide to Creating Crystal Essences for Abundant
Well-Being, Environmental Healing and Astral Magic
ISBN: 978-1-78904-052-4 (Paperback) £17.99 $29.95

Introduction: Time to let go

Let them look to the past, but let them also look to the future; let them look to the land of their ancestors, but let them look also to the land of their children.
Wilfrid Laurier

Listen to the voices, feelings, sights and experiences of our ancestors. Their lives, joys and fears are within us. In that way, they are with us always.
Steve Hammons[1]

As a karmic astrologer and longtime chronicler of the soul's journey, I recognised sometime ago that we cannot make the predicted shift from the Age of Pisces to the 'new' Age of Aquarius whilst dragging the past behind us. Healing must precede evolution. We need to do a massive clearing first. We all have stuff we need to revisit, dust off, and let go: transgenerational and ancestral in addition to karmic and individual. Wounds that need to be healed: personal, familial, planetary and humanitarian. Beliefs and attitudes that need to be examined and reframed where necessary. Souls that need to be reclaimed, repaired and reintegrated. Timelines that need to be unsnagged and realigned. Soul learnings that need to be recognised and honoured.

Healing

In the context of this book, healing means letting go of the past, transmuting and returning to balance on every level. It does not imply a cure.

There's a racial, collective and cosmic aspect to this clearing. What we do now will benefit the generations to come – and free up those that have passed. I briefly covered some of those aspects in *Crystal Prescriptions volume 5*, but this present book goes into greater depth, especially as to the underlying mechanism of both personal and ancestral karmic issues. The more we understand how these can be conveyed across the generations, the more options we have for a healing intervention. Fortunately there are efficient crystal tools to assist in unravelling the layers.

Timelines

Time is not linear. It is circular and complex, interwoven like a spider's web – and does not exist as we know it once you step beyond the confines of Earth. Timelines are strings of lives that can best be visualised as 'theme' threads that can attract or repel each other and interweave, carrying imprints and blockages from other lives and different timeframes (see illustration on page 185). Timelines carried by those with whom we have an energetic interaction, previous life or transgeneration connections, can quickly mesh together, entangling the timelines and pulling us back into old, outworn patterns, as can our own past life timelines and unfinished business.

Man did not weave the web of life. He is merely a strand in it. Whatever he does to the web, he does to himself.
Chief Seattle

Other lives/past lives

The previous lives that a soul (or a soul family) has lived upon the Earth and in other planes of existence.

Compassionate self-care

The fact that 'the past' needs healing does not mean that you need to berate yourself – or the ancestors – for having 'got it wrong'. It's all part of an ongoing learning process. We all need to take responsibility for the remedial work, however: working for ourselves *and* on behalf of the ancestors and future generations. It is not a matter of rightness or wrongness, and especially not of fault or blame. We need to do this with compassion, forgiveness and unconditional love. It is a question of soul expansion *and* of returning our soul and our ancestral line to a state of realignment with our true being whilst incorporating all that has been learnt. Only when we individually make such a shift can the whole benefit. And, when doing this work, it is important that we do not regard ourselves as damaged victims, abusers or refusers. We need to recognise that we are eternal souls who have undertaken a human journey in order to learn or to serve and contribute to the whole, and who are now making a shift to a more evolved way of being. We are expanding our awareness and realising that we are more than our body, more than our karmic or ancestral history. At our core, we are pure spirit consciousness and, when we come from that place, healing flows and evolution occurs. As Hareesh puts it:

> *It's this simple: you cannot heal the 'broken self' as long as you believe that you are it. Or you can, but it's ridiculously difficult. By contrast, if you wake up to and become centered in your real nature, then you can lovingly address any misalignments in the body-mind… If you're willing to do the work of integration, every layer of your being becomes permeated with the powerful energy of awakeness. You start to then embody that awakeness, which is beneficial to all beings. If you don't do the work of integration, even if you're centered in your divine core,*

you're not really benefitting anyone else.
Christopher Wallis (also known as Hareesh)[2]

This is where crystals can be so helpful. They embody that 'true nature' in its perfect form and facilitate returning our own awareness to that unbroken state. Crystals themselves may have been broken, blasted or dispossessed of their land, but they have within them the innate ability to return to that state of energetic perfection no matter what, and bring you to that place also.

Ancestral line

The ancestral line carries your family history. The beliefs, experiences, dramas, traumas, dominant emotions and assigned roles that stretch back into eternity. Not merely physical DNA, the ancestral line includes subtle energetic DNA and 'junk DNA'. It is an energetic web encompassing past, present and future – and beyond.

The lineage story

In addition to our own karma and early life experiences, we are imbued with ancestral memories, attitudes and beliefs that are not personal. These pass down the family line, carried in the genetic memory, rarely being re-examined for relevance or effect. For the most part, we've forgotten who we really are at our core – and why we are here on Earth. We have become disconnected from our overall soulplan and our spiritual roots – which have nothing to do with religious orientation. We may not feel we belong. There are those who remember 'not being from here' and yearn to return to the stars, or to being a disembodied spiritual being. Some even remember being crystals.

Numerous people in the modern world live with a sense of being 'the dispossessed', 'the exiles', 'the incomer', and do not feel part of the land on which they now reside. They feel rootless, or look back longingly to a 'homeland' that may have only existed many generations previously. Or perhaps never at all. Even if they have adapted to their modern environment, their parents and grandparents – in incarnation or out – may still yearn for the mythic 'promised land'. It has become part of the lineage story, whether actually factually true or not. The Jewish and Irish races are a prime example of this, but millions of refugees fled from wars, natural disasters or famine, or made the choice to be economic migrants over the centuries. It is deeply embedded – and not always at a conscious level. However, there can also be a positive side to the story if the strengths, soul learnings and survival strategies of previous generations can be integrated (see page 227).

We inherit these ancestral yearnings along with so many other patterns and, all too unconsciously, live them out time and again. They are carried in our 'junk DNA' (more of that later) and karmic imprints and 'engrams', and we replay them until cleared. The story usually fits with our own karma. But it's carried in the ancestral DNA and the collective may also require clearing. Someone has to do it. Many people who are in incarnation now came in with the intention of being lineage breakers: healers for the ancestral line and the collective, in addition to the personal karmic past. Some of us may also be hampered by soul loss, parts of our soul left in other lives or other dimensions. Or we may have an ancestral or other spirit attachment, a hitchhiker who, for whatever reason, has hooked into our energy field and is attempting to influence our actions. We may need to retrieve, cleanse and reintegrate our soul. Crystals are only too happy to facilitate this.

Karma

Cause and effect. A soul-growth tool. Karma is an ongoing process that can create beneficial or detrimental results in every moment but cannot be judged from the standpoint of one life. Never fixed or unyielding, karma is fluid and can be transmuted.

It's up to you

I am alive............and it begins with me......!
Michael Vincent

If you're on Earth right now, you've volunteered to be part of the karmic clean-up squad, readying the world for a consciousness shift. Whether you know it or not, you're a lineage breaker. Sort your own karma, dump your baggage, detox your ancestral line; retrieve transgenerational strengths and soul learning; reintegrate your soul, find your divine roots, and the collective can only benefit. As will you. It's time to create a more positive future for everyone. Now!

Lineage breakers

Lineage breakers incarnate to break the ancestral chain and start a new, more positive pattern.

Crystal facilitators

Some extraordinary new crystals have appeared to help us to do this work. Quickly, easily and without having to relive the trauma and dramas of the ancestors, or our own karmic history. Ancestralite, for instance, is the perfect crystal for the ancestral line as it goes back to the beginning, heals the past and brings the soul insights forward, but without the traumatic underpinnings. We can 'put our soul back together' and integrate the ancestral learning with new, more positive programmes installed. With the assistance of these amazing crystals, and some old favourites, we can heal far back into the ancestral tree and our karmic past, projecting the healing forward into the future so that the generations to come can have the benefit of our soul and ancestral wisdom without the family baggage.

Soul

Soul is ancient, immortal, indestructible – although it may fragment and leave particles of itself in other lives and other dimensions. The whole soul rarely incarnates in one life or one place at a time.

How crystals can help

Many of the biochemical processes within the body involve exchanges of physical energy, but these grosser forms of energy are not what I take the terms healing energy and subtle energy to mean. Rather, the latter are like the activity of a conductor of an orchestra or the choreographer of a ballet that integrates and coordinates into one cohesive movement all the bio-chemical and energy processes of the body.

F. David Peat

Crystals heal holistically – that is to say, they work at a causal level on the whole person. I would liken a crystal to the conductor or choreographer of which David Peat speaks.

Crystals, despite their apparently solid appearance,

are actually thousands of molecules whizzing around in a stable holding pattern. That pattern is more coherent than anything in the human body. The human body too is held together by energetic forces but the human bioenergy field is inherently unstable. Place a crystal in that field, however, and the energies 'entrain'. That is to say, the stable field corrects the unstable one and brings it into balance. But crystals go further than this. They can expand the human energy field so that the molecules 'move apart' and release any detrimental pattern or information that is being held in that field. They release timelines, soul contracts, vows, outdated programs and the like that are still running in the background in the same way as occurs in computers. These programs slow you down, pulling you back into your own karmic or ancestral past. But run a virus check, defrag your computer, remove outdated programmes, and the system frees up. A new program can then be imprinted with a higher resonance crystal.

Soul contract

An agreement willingly – or unwillingly – made in a previous life, or in the interlife before the present incarnation, that one soul would interact with another in a specific way. Or, an agreement that is carried over from a previous life, or a previous interlife plan, but which has not been reconsidered before incarnation. Soul contracts can be positive and constructive, or destructive. Soul contracts that are not completed in one life may be carried over to another.

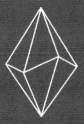

Part I
The Basics

Do, please, read this section even if you are an
experienced crystal worker. It may well contain
concepts with which you are unfamiliar as it includes
foundational material and healing interventions that
are applicable across more than one section of
the book.

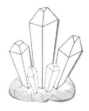

Safe working practices:
the four essentials

As the late Alan Watts put it:
Reality is only a Rorschach ink-blot, you know.

All the healing and clearing work in this book is assisted by your own energy and your space being as protected, balanced, grounded and clear as possible. Some of the soul work is challenging and best done with the assistance of a qualified practitioner. But there are times when emergency work is required, and much of the ancestral and karmic healing and clearing can be undertaken with the invaluable assistance of crystals and your own common sense. However, never, ever, attempt this work in a space that is not safe or when your chakras are seriously out of balance, or your auric field compromised. If so, you may be open to psychic invasion or spirit attachment that will exacerbate the situation rather than heal it. Crystals quickly create a protected space around you so keep one or two about your person just in case. Grounding is also essential for clarity and successful completion of the work. Familiarising yourself with basic practices and concepts now will make the healing work much more fruitful and effective.

1. Screen yourself...

Crystals are excellent for protecting and screening your energy when working. Wearing a Labradorite over your higher heart chakra (above the thymus, centre chest), for instance, screens external energies and creates an interface between the internal and external worlds. This allows you to be intuitively aware of what is going on with the ancestral, soul or karmic line – or yourself – without getting sucked into the issues. Healer's Gold works in the same way to create an interface but can also create a firewall when appropriate. Placing Yellow Labradorite, Lapis Lazuli or Apophyllite on the third eye helps you to be more intuitively aware of subtle energies and to communicate with Spirit and the ancestors. You don't need big shiny crystals for this; small, raw pieces will do. Rhomboid Selenite is the crystal to go to if your third eye has been sealed in the past. It clears prohibitions and restrictions imposed prior to incarnation or in childhood.

If you feel energetically depleted when with a particular person, or have a constant ache under your left armpit, then you need to pay attention to your spleen chakra (see page 37 and *Crystal Prescriptions 4 and 5* for in-depth information on this chakra). This is where the energy vampires hook in and suck out your energy.

Fortunately a Green Aventurine or Flint quickly disconnects these cords, and Green Aventurine, Fluorite or Jade over the spleen chakra protects you from taking on 'stuff' from other people or having them leech your energy. If you then get a pain under the right armpit, this is the result of an energy vampire becoming angry at having its power source cut off. Tape a piece of Gaspeite, Tugtupite or Bloodstone over the site and leave in place for several days until the message is received that you will not be giving away any more of your energy. This works particularly well for energy vampires who are still among the living, or those who are dead but not departed.

2. Keep your space safe

Your space can be protected by creating a grid with Black Tourmaline, Smoky Quartz, Labradorite or Selenite. Three stones arranged in a triangle work well, as do crystals in each corner of the room. If you put a few drops of Petaltone Z14 (see Resources) on the stones, the energies will be cleansed to very high levels and it will transmute everything that is released within the space. The grid then maintains the clean, safe space for several months. This works well for moving on spirits trapped in a particular environment. (See *Crystal Prescriptions volume 5* and *Good Vibrations: Psychic Protection, Energy Enhancement and Space Clearing* for additional assistance.) A few drops of Petaltone Astral Clear on a clear Quartz point is invaluable for moving on spirits that are attached to a place or to an object (see page 212). Ask the crystal to send the spirit to the light, or from whence it came if it belongs in another dimension. Place the crystal in the room or environment and leave it overnight.

Safe space

An area, large or small, which is protected and cleansed so that nothing negative or untoward can penetrate or interfere with what goes on in that space.

---

3. Keep your crystals clean

Crystals work hard on your behalf, drawing off toxic energy and transmuting detrimental patterns. They absorb karmic dross and ancestral blight, and can act as a repository for soul parts undergoing healing and assist with reintegration. It is a matter of good sense to regularly cleanse and recharge them as otherwise the cycle may repeat itself. (See pages 123–125.)

4. And finally, ground yourself!

In order to be effective when using crystals for healing, and in order to gain maximum benefit from crystal healing, you need to be centred and grounded. Grounding is a term that means you are solidly anchored in the present, with a certain inner stillness, a feeling of being secure, in control of yourself and alert.

Simon Lilly, *Crystals and Crystal Healing*

Before beginning any work on cleansing karma and the ancestral line, or soul healing, it is essential to ground and stabilise yourself. This can be done through the earthy chakras at your feet, knees and belly with the assistance of Flint, Hematite or other grounding stones. You can then open the higher chakras and safely explore the past. (You will find an illustration of all the chakras on page 25.)

Symptoms of ungroundedness

Check out these symptoms. Tick more than three or four and you definitely need to ground yourself.

- Mental confusion/inability to concentrate
- Inability to handle the everyday world
- Life and home are cluttered
- Eyes are blank: 'no one home'
- Spaced out, vague and unfocused
- Difficulty in motivating yourself
- Leaving everything to the last minute, but not living in the moment
- Always running late
- Dizziness or 'woozy headed'
- Clumsiness and dyspraxia – you often bump into things
- Appearing to float several inches above the floor
- Sugar craving and a desire for junk food
- Constantly hungry but food doesn't satisfy
- Falling asleep while meditating

- Car or electrical equipment breaks down regularly
- Irritability without due cause
- Insomnia and restless sleep
- Unwanted out-of-body experiences
- Sense of looking down on yourself from above
- Body feels heavy and 'alien'
- Emotional and highly over-reactive
- Constantly exhausted
- Great ideas or plans that never come to fruition
- Belching or breaking wind frequently
- Anxiety or unease with no apparent cause
- Displaying the same symptoms as someone you were just with
- Mood changes suddenly when passing a stranger or entering a room
- Bank account is frequently in the red

Creating your grounding root

This simple grounding root exercise anchors you to the planet, re-energizes you from the Earth, and allows freedom of movement in order to reach higher or further dimensions of consciousness, to journey inwards or back into the past, and to safely access the Akashic Record. Remember to cleanse and dedicate your crystals before you begin the exercise (see pages 123–125).

- *Cleanse the aura and chakras with Flint and/or Anandalite (if you don't have Anandalite or the other crystals you can use the cards in* The Crystal Wisdom

Healing Oracle *pack).*

- *Stand with your feet slightly apart, well balanced on your knees and hips. Feet flat on the floor. Place a Flint, Eye of the Storm (Judy's Jasper), Graphic Smoky Quartz, Hematite, Smoky Quartz, Smoky Elestial Quartz or other grounding stone at your feet.*
- *Picture the earth star chakra about a foot beneath your feet opening like the petals of a water lily.*
- *Place your hands just below your navel (tummy button) with fingertips touching and palms out towards the hips.*
- *Picture roots spreading across your belly, into your hips and then down through your legs and out of your feet to meet in the grounding stone.*
- *The two roots twine together and pass down through the earth star and the Gaia gateway, going deep into the Earth. They pass through the outer mantle, down past the solid crust and deep into the molten magma.*
- *When the entwined roots have passed through the magma, they reach the big iron crystal ball at the centre of the planet.*
- *The roots hook themselves around this ball, holding you firmly in incarnation and helping you to be grounded in incarnation.*
- *Energy and protection can flow up this root to keep you energized and safe.*
- *Allow the roots to pass up from the earth star through your feet, up your legs and the knee chakras and into your hips. At your hips the roots move across to meet in*

the base chakra and from there to the sacral and the dantien just below your navel. The energy that flows up from the centre of the Earth can be stored in the dantien.

Note: Whenever you are in an area of disturbed earth energy, or a place where you have traumatic previous life or genealogical connections, protect your earth star and Gaia gateway chakras by visualising a large protective crystal all around them. The root will still be able to pass down to the centre of the Earth to bring powerful energy to support you, and the crystal will help to transmute and stabilise the negative energy. A virtual crystal can work equally well when visualised with intent, but placing an actual crystal here intensifies the effect.

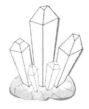

The chakra system and its place in transgenerational and karmic issues

The chakras are multi-layered, multidimensional vortexes of subtle energy that radiate several feet out all around your physical body. Linkage points between the physical and subtle energy bodies, they are metaphysical energy portals, rather than physical, but they are essential to our efficient functioning in the world and to raising consciousness. Chakras mediate how much you take in from the world around you, and govern your response to that outer world. Loosely speaking, the chakras below the waist are primarily physical, although they can affect the endocrine glands and from that personality. Those in the upper torso are aligned to emotional functioning and engrams that can create psychosomatic conditions, as can those in the head that function on a mental and intuitive basis but which may have physical repercussions. Both the past life chakras (behind the ears) and the causal vortex (above and to the side of the head) hold karmic and ancestral memories. Chakras above and around the head are spiritual connection points and the soma chakra (mid-hairline) and the heart seed chakra (below the breastbone) are both points where the soul and spirit attach.

All the chakras can hold and replay ancestral and karmic themes.

Each of the chakras has specific ancestral or karmic links and carries inter- or cross-generational themes. They also link to particular levels of karma: personal, ancestral, collective and cosmic (see page 164). When blocked (closed) and blown (too open), the chakras replay karmic or ancestral issues and reflect inherited transgenerational themes. In addition to chakra issues acquired in the present life, you may be born with blocked or blown chakras if the predisposition is carried by the matriarchal or your own karmic line. Or, they may be created in utero by your mother's experience and emotions. Issues and transgenerational themes can be resolved by placing appropriate crystals on to the chakra or navel to rebalance it.

Transgenerational themes

A transgenerational (that is, crossing the generations) theme can arise from a single, potent act of trauma, oft-repeated traumas, or from inherited intransigent attitudes, beliefs and events. Transgenerational themes reverberate and are played out through several generations experiencing the same type of issue or dis-ease. Themes are passed down the ancestral line encoded in the 'junk DNA' (see page 83) and may be expressed through the psoas or 'soul' muscle (see page 76).

What blocks a chakra?

There are many reasons why a chakra may become blocked or blown. Old traumas, toxicity, close-mindedness and fixed beliefs, emotional pain and physical injuries can all contribute as can karmic imprints and engrams. These blockages are not merely personal. They can also be passed along the ancestral line. They become an energetic pattern, or engram, that is imprinted into the relevant chakra and subtle energy bodies at a very deep level. However, one of the major causes of blocked or blown chakras is past life or ancestral issues that have been carried over into the present life or brought in via the DNA, and which are reactivated by present life experiences. The A–Z Directory covers crystals to remedy a wide range of these causes, as well as the addictions and emotional blockages that can result.

These issues are imprinted in the karmic and ancestral subtle energy bodies, in 'junk DNA', and the past life and

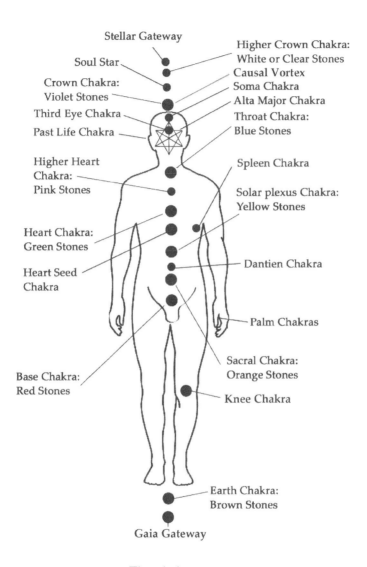

The chakra system

causal vortex chakras. The layers may need to be peeled back gently over a period of time until the core issue is reached. It can then be released and the energy transmuted. When ancestral clearing or detaching a spirit on behalf of someone other than yourself who is not present, rather than using yourself as a surrogate, which could work well or could leave you vulnerable if you are not fully grounded and protected, you can lay appropriate crystals on the chakra diagram on page 25.

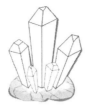

Karmic themes in the chakras

Gaia Gateway

Location: About an arm's length beneath your feet, below the earth star.

Karmic level: Ancestral, personal and collective.

A higher resonance of the earth star, this chakra carries the karma of the planet and the wisdom of the ancestors. The karma held here is ancestral and collective. This chakra connects your soul to the soul and spirit of the planet, Gaia, and to Mother Earth herself. When your Gaia gateway is open and functioning at optimum, you are aware of being a particle of a sacred whole, part of the energy system of the Earth and All That Is. When balanced and open, this chakra helps you to protect yourself from spirit attachment and lower energies.

When this chakra is blown it leads to extreme sensitivity to Earth changes. Overwhelming memories of past disasters may be present. Being in incarnation, and especially being in a physical body, is challenging and there is no ability to remain stable during periods of energetic uplift. When this chakra is blocked there is an inability to ground and connect with higher energies.

Karmic and ancestral issues: Accepting or rejecting being an equal part of humanity and at-one-ness with the whole cosmos. Plundering the planet's resources. The karma or ancestral issues are ones of disconnection from the Earth as a sacred, living being, replaying or making restitution for greed and over-utilisation of the planet's resources with disregard for others who share the planet as a karmic or ancestral pattern.

Earth Star

Location: About a foot beneath the feet.

Karmic level: Ancestral, collective and personal.

The earth star chakra connects you to the Earth's core as well as its meridians. This chakra is a place of safety and regeneration. Without it, you may have only a toehold in incarnation, and be physically and psychologically ungrounded. When this chakra is functioning well you are grounded and comfortable in incarnation. You operate well in everyday reality and will be open to clearing karma for the ancestors and the collective.

If your earth star is blown you will lack grounding and have no connection to the planet or awareness of being part of a greater overall system. Or, paradoxically, you may be overly concerned for the planet with insufficient attention given to your own body. An out of balance earth star easily picks up adverse environmental factors such as previous events, geopathic stress and toxic pollutants. Earth star blockages or disruptions replay previous

discomfort in a physical body and a sense of not belonging on the planet.

Karmic and ancestral issues: The karma held here covers racial identity, power, security and survival, dealing with everyday reality; misusing the resources of the planet, or lacking the resources to sustain life. With little body awareness, the ancestral inheritance is feelings of helplessness and alienation, accompanied by an inability to function practically in the world.

Knee

Location: Behind and through the knees, like a flat disc on which the body rests.

Karmic level: Ancestral, collective and personal.

The knee chakras ensure you are flexible and able to adapt to changing circumstances. They may suffer a left-right imbalance. Generally speaking, the left knee represents the matriarchal line. The feminine, yin aspect, that is receptive, emotional and intuitive. The right knee represents the patriarchal line. It is the yang aspect that is factual, practical, managerial and outgoing. A blown knee chakra constantly meets problems with authority, authority figures and bureaucracy – a replaying of past issues. There is a need to be in control. Arrogant superiority is common. This is the person who thinks he, or she, 'knows best' and demands subservience from others. Control-freakery is common as is jumping from the frying pan into the fire.

Chronic fear and feelings of inferiority and consequent subservience are reflected in blocked knee chakras. Unhealthy dependent and controlling relationships including 'codependency', constant challenge by others or difficulties in intimacy and closeness are common. There is an expectation of lack of basic sustenance, materially, nutritionally and spiritually. The soul feels empty.

Karmic and ancestral issues: Authority, inflexibility, servility, servitude, fear of change especially death, and right use of willpower. The karma and ancestral inheritance is to do with the ability to nurture and support yourself and manifest what you need on a day to day basis.

Base

Location: Base of your spine, tailbone, coccyx, perineum.

Karmic level: Ancestral and personal.

Your base chakra is linked to your connection to Earth and to your body. It represents both your ancestry, home and place in the world. When it functions well you are connected to your core. The base chakra is the area of the will to survive and the ability to make things happen. This is where you discover yourself as an individual and take responsibility for yourself. It is where you recognise the tribe to which you belong and where you feel safe. When this chakra is functioning well, you trust the universe.

The sexual karma carried here may be personal or ancestral. Imbalances lead to sexual disturbances and feelings of stuckness, anger, impotence and frustration – and the inability to let go. When this chakra is racing flat out it is easy to become sexually obsessed, continually seeking satisfaction 'out there' rather than making an inner connection and developing personality traits that will sustain you. This can lead to alcohol, drug and other addictive or comfort-seeking behaviour – which will be a repeating pattern arising from a sense of lack in the past. You will be floaty, ungrounded, and may experience uncontrolled out-of-body experiences, dark sexual fantasies and vivid dreams. When this chakra is blocked, it replays past impotence – and may become physical. Lacking bioenergetic balance, you may be unwilling to accept your connection to the Earth, feeling uncomfortable in your physical body and seeking escape.

Karmic and ancestral issues: Creativity, basic survival instincts and security, abuse, sexual mores and attitudes passed down through the family. Previous vows and soul contracts. The karma will be that of feelings of isolation and alienation and, at the extreme, to fantasies of self-destruction. You may be stuck in fight or flight mode.

Sacral

Location: About a hand's breadth below your waist.

Karmic and ancestral level: Personal and ancestral.

This creative chakra holds your core energy and reflects your energetic inheritance. When this chakra is working well you experience yourself as a dynamic agent of change in your life. If it is blocked, you cannot experience yourself as a potent sexual being. You may feel shut off from nurturing and sharing, or replay jealousy and possessiveness.

If this chakra is blown, you may be subjected to overwhelming sexual urges and attract disembodied spirits who thrive on sexual energy. This chakra affects how easily you express your sexuality and how you feel about relationships: frustration may occur at all levels. It may also replay parenting issues and the connection to your family. The sacral chakra is where 'hooks' from other people may make themselves felt, particularly from previous sexual encounters. Blockages reflect a family embargo on feeling good and worthy. When this chakra is blocked you may experience powerlessness, chronic lower back or pelvic pain, or gynaecological problems that replay past issues.

Karmic and ancestral issues: Creativity, passion, potency, fertility, previous soul contracts, independence. The karma and ancestral inheritance carried here has a great deal to do with how you handle your immediate environment and matters such as money, career and authority figures.

The Dantien

Location: Two–three fingers' breadth below the navel (above the sacral).

Karmic and ancestral level: Personal, ancestral and collective.

The dantien is one of the most powerful places for

transmuting timelines and karma carried in the spaces between the molecules of the physical body and in the 'junk DNA'. An adjunct to the sacral chakra and the point of balance for the physical body, the dantien is where life force is stored and your body earthed. A disconnection here means that you do not feel like you belong on the Earth and you are powerless to control your life. Ancestral or karmic issues take over. When working positively, this chakra is where you become centred around your inner core. When you are connected to your core, you not only have more physical energy as you are not affected by life's ups and downs, but you are also more emotionally stable and better able to resist stress. You are not easily thrown off balance. Nor are you open to manipulation by others. When it is blocked, you may easily be pushed around or manipulated by other people, despite feeling that you are in control. When the dantien is full of power, you have inner resources to draw on. You are literally power-full. When it is functioning well you are energized, stable and well grounded. If the dantien is too open, you are ungrounded, labile, frenetic and energy is constantly drained.

Karmic and ancestral issues: Dispossession, alienation, powerlessness, stability, power, self-assertion, manipulation. The karmic and ancestral patterns replayed here centre around power or abuse and misuse of power. The autoimmune system cannot function, with resultant dis-ease that reflects your ancestral or karmic inheritance.

The Navel ('Tummy button')

Location: Centre line, just below the waist.

Karmic level: Ancestral, matriarchal.

The navel ('tummy button') is not a chakra as such but it is where the connection to the mother and the matriarchal line is strongest pre-birth, with nutrients – physical or subtle – having to pass through the umbilical cord. It is, therefore, a potent place for ancestral line connection and the passage of transgenerational messages, both via DNA and matriarchal imperatives. The placenta, which is designed to be a life-support system for the unborn child, may in fact carry a toxic soup of all the mother's emotions and traumas. If the psychic umbilical cord is not cut, the mother and her demands dominate. The navel can be an extremely vulnerable area. It is known as the tummy 'button' for good, although probably largely unconscious, reasons. It can be the trigger point for ancestral memories to surface, especially of fear and trauma. Working with crystals around the navel to expand and release subtle memory patterns can be highly effective. Particularly as energy gaps, rips and tears can be present at this site in the subtle energy bodies as well as in the physical. Anandalite, Ancestralite, Cradle of Life (Humankind), Lemurian Seed, Menalite, Preseli Bluestone and Celtic Healer Quartz are particularly effective for working around the navel along with other ancestral line stones (see page 281 in the A–Z Directory).

Karmic and ancestral issues: Receiving and giving love, safety and security, self-worth, alienation and acceptance, fitting into society and the environment, power: dominance and submission.

To clear matriarchal and intrauterine imprints from the navel chakra

- *Open your grounding root (see page 19), lie down and place a grounding stone slightly to one side of your feet, opposite the causal vortex chakra (see page 25) to anchor it.*
- *Place Anandalite, Blue Kyanite, Selenite or other crystal on the causal vortex chakra.*
- *Place a Menalite, Cradle of Life or other navel chakra stone on your navel.*
- *Place your hands in your groin creases.*
- *Lie still for five to fifteen minutes.*
- *When complete, remove the causal vortex chakra crystal and replace it with the grounding stone to close the chakra.*
- *Remove the navel chakra stone.*
- *Ground yourself thoroughly once more.*

Solar Plexus

Location: Hand's breadth above the waist.

Karmic level: Personal and ancestral.

The solar plexus is the place of digestion on all levels. It acts as a point of equilibrium between your present soul purpose and your past karma so that previous learning is applied wisely. When blocked or blown, the karma stored in this chakra can lead to taking on other people's feelings and problems, especially where these reflect your own past issues or feelings that were taboo in the family. You may be overwhelmed by your own unrecognised emotions. Emotional 'hooks' from other people can be found here. You may endlessly try to fix in other people what you would be better attending to in yourself. You could be prey to wild intuitions, premonitions of doom and a paranoid suspicion that the whole world is out to get you. When this chakra is blocked you will be unable to empathise or share your own feelings with others – although you may still be overwhelmed by theirs. There will be a sense of inferiority and a tendency to cling too tightly or to push other people away. Intimacy and sharing is impossible when this chakra is blocked.

Karmic and ancestral issues: Emotional communication or lack of it. The solar plexus is where emotions and karmic and ancestral inheritance is stored and it can have a profound psychosomatic effect. Feelings and blocked emotions are reflected in inherited and personal dis-eases. 'Illness as theatre' replays out the emotional story in the symptoms. Another person may easily become entrapped in the family saga as the 'care-giver', scapegoat or identified patient.

Spleen

Location: A hand's breadth below the left armpit extending down towards the waist, back and front.

Karmic level: Racial, personal and ancestral.

The spleen chakra is an energy portal and, when the chakra is wide open, other people can draw on your energy, leaving you depleted. You will pick up other people's feelings, especially anger and irritation which can lead to physical pain. You may remain connected to anyone with whom you have had close contact *even if this was in another life*. People can easily take advantage of you, manipulating and coercing you into self-destructive actions that are not for your highest good. Your body may well turn in to attack itself leading to autoimmune diseases. Uncontrollable anger is common when this chakra is blown as you unconsciously rebel against being subtly manipulated or vampirised.

With ancestral karma replayed in this chakra, you may feel rootless, purposeless, exhausted and manipulated, powerless. You may well have anger issues, but find it difficult to express your anger. You may also suffer constant irritation, some of which goes back to unresolved past life issues. As with the blown chakra, your body may turn in to attack itself. Intimacy with others is impossible when this chakra is locked shut.

Karmic and ancestral issues: Self-protection and empowerment.

To cleanse and protect the spleen chakra (spleen chakra release)

- *Cleanse your spleen chakra by spiralling out a Quartz point, Green Aventurine, Flint, raw Charoite or Rainbow Mayanite under your left armpit to clear any hooks or energetic connections from the chakra.*
- *To protect the chakra after tie cutting, tape a Tantalite, Green Aventurine, Green Fluorite or Jade crystal over the spleen chakra, or wear one on a long chain so that it reaches to the end of your breastbone level with the chakra.*
- *Picture a three-dimensional green pyramid extending down from your armpit to your waist, front and back to protect the spleen.*
- *If the area under your right armpit then begins to ache, tape a piece of Gaspeite, Tugtupite or Bloodstone over the site and leave in place for several days until the message is received that you will not be giving away any more of your energy. You can also picture a red three-dimensional pyramid protecting this area.*

Palm

Location: The palms of the hands.

Karmic level: Mainly personal but may hold ancestral issues.

Powerful sensors, hands assist you to interact with the world on an energetic level. They are intimately connected with your ability to receive and to generate, manifest and *actualise*. If too open, you may constantly try to assist others but in an over-the-top, extreme, martyred way. When blown, extreme touchiness is common. There is an inability to receive, including a refusal to ask for help or accept it when offered. Lack of connection with the world and with other people may result in antisocial behaviour. At the extreme, this becomes psychopathic or sociopathic. Unsociability includes refusing to share as well as to assist others in times of need.

Karmic and ancestral issues: Giving and receiving, grasping greed, numbness. Closed off and withdrawn from society, antisocial but paradoxically needy without knowing the reason why.

Heart Seed

Location: Over the xiphoid process, at the tip of breastbone below the heart chakra.

Karmic level: Cosmic, collective, ancestral and personal.

The heart seed creates a connection to who you really are. It helps you to recall the reason for incarnation, encouraging you to be in spiritual service to humanity. However, it may also replay ancestral imperatives around service, slavery and servility until these are released. Opening this chakra connects you to your soul purpose and shows how it fits into the overall divine plan. It also assists in renegotiating a past-its-sell-by-date soul purpose or soul contract. This chakra facilitates activating the karmic tools you have available, the soul lessons you have already learned. When the heart seed chakra is blown, heart energy and compassion cannot be integrated or expended appropriately. It can result in depletion and exhaustion from being overly compassionate, giving without consideration as to whether this is necessary or appropriate. It can result in spiritual interference with another person's journey and life lessons. It can also result in the spiritual martyr who feels hard done by. Or, playing the victim or rescuer, as others take advantage. If the heart seed is blocked, you are cut off from your purpose in incarnating.

Karmic and ancestral issues: Victim-martyr-saviour-rescuer scenarios, achieving unity consciousness, spiritual purpose, service and religion versus spirituality, soul remembrance.

Heart

Location: Centre of chest, towards base of breastbone.

Karmic level: Personal, ancestral and collective.

The heart chakra is the core of your being. It is the site of the bonds you make with other people, your relationships, and your interaction with the wider worlds around you. When this chakra is blown you are ruled by your emotions, reacting rather than responding. Happiness, sadness, anger, grief, neediness are overwhelming. Feelings and emotions are not processed, and may be projected out to the world and perceived in the actions of others. This chakra has a strong connection to the past life chakras and previous life heartache may make itself felt, leading to a lack of trust. This chakra is vulnerable and can easily become codependent, needy and manipulative – and conditional. 'Too much love' is common, indiscriminately pouring out sickly sweet love to cover self-perceived feelings of inadequacy, lack of self-worth and wanting, no matter how subconsciously, to make reparation for the past. This is the person who serves in order to be perceived as being a good person. But, in relationships, will always be the giver, not the receiver. Balance may be lacking. Covering up or apologising for others, and constantly forgiving, leads to hanging on at all costs to a relationship that will most certainly not be for the highest good.

Intimacy is a huge challenge when this chakra is closed off. With this chakra blocked, you feel under-valued and misunderstood. Feelings of inferiority, a sense of being unlovable and unloved, replays a fear of rejection and a desperate desire not to be alone, but those very feelings push other people away. Or, you push people away before they can leave you. Equally, you may settle for abusive or collusive relationships in order to satisfy the need not to be alone.

This chakra holds on to past life pain and heartbreak. When blocked, it results in an inability to forgive yourself or those who have hurt you – and you will have a hard time trusting people because your experiences 'confirm' that what you fear is true will come about, again and again. It is a self-fulfilling prophecy. You set extremely high standards for yourself – and others –

creating a self-perpetuating loop whereby you are too hard on yourself, feel a failure and experience both guilt and self-hatred. Energy from a blocked heart chakra can be subverted to the spleen, where it is experienced as anger attacking seemingly from outside. It may also be bounced back into the base and sacral chakra leading to sexual obsession especially when meeting an old love once again.

Karmic and ancestral issues: Love and intimacy in all its forms, possessiveness, perception of being loved. The challenge is to overcome the karmic or ancestral fear that 'there will never be enough love'.

Higher Heart (Thymus)

Location: Over the thymus gland, between the heart and the throat.

Karmic level: Personal, ancestral and cosmic.

This chakra governs the physical and psychic immune systems, and how you protect yourself. The thymus gland is the first gland to develop in the uterus and, therefore, is a core component of how your body functions *in utero*, governing which genetic potential gets switched on in the 'junk DNA'. Connected to ancestral DNA and to the past life patterning, if this chakra is blocked the physical body replays blockages and engrams through a compromised immune system and dis-eases.

Karmic and ancestral issues: Paranoia, spiritual disconnection, grief, need, a psychic vampire.

Throat

Location: The centre of the throat.

Karmic level: Personal and ancestral.

This chakra is all about communication and it can affect how valued and nurtured you feel. It is where you express yourself, including strongly felt feelings and emotions that come from the heart or solar plexus chakra as well as thoughts. If it is blocked and there is no outlet for these feelings and thoughts, it can lead to psychosomatic dis-ease. It can also lead to speaking what you think others wish to hear rather than being honest and sharing your heartfelt truth. You may feel that you have no right to express an opinion.

When this chakra is blocked, your truth cannot be expressed. You may not be able to stand up for yourself and may well be bullied. You may suffer from extreme shyness or believe that other people will not value, or may reject, what you have to say. You were probably told as a child that children should be seen and not heard. There will be a great fear of being judged and inability to verbally defend or explain yourself. The world may be experienced as hostile or prejudging and so you reject it. A deficient or distorted throat chakra may also lead to egotism and judgementalism because other people's self-expression is feared, overruled or disregarded.

Karmic and ancestral issues: Communication, speaking truth.

Past Life

Location: Along the bony ridge behind the ears.

Karmic level: Personal, ancestral, collective.

The past life chakras are where you store the memories of your previous lives. This elongated dual chakra links to the karmic blueprint, which has soul wounds, physical and emotional, from the past embedded in it. This may create psychosomatic dis-ease or actual physical disease, which is carried through engrams or subtle memory traces. An engram is a mental image that records an experience containing pain, unconsciousness and a real or fancied threat to survival. Activating these chakras could bring up many memories to be released, but they may also help you to reconnect to soul gifts that you have developed in the past.

When these chakras are wide open, there is no filter and no understanding of what is past and what is present. Past life experiences constantly impinge on the present to the extent that there may be emotional or psychiatric disturbances. Deep fear, paranoia and other manifestations are common. Emotional baggage and unfinished business constantly sabotage daily life. When the chakras are blown, you will feel unsafe and subconsciously overwhelmed by past life memories of trauma, violent death and fears – even when these are at an, unrecognised, unconscious level. This leaves the way open for past life personas, soul fragments and thought forms to attach or re-manifest.

Blockages here mean that you are stuck in the past

and cannot move forward. You may well be repeating your own past life patterns or recreating ancestral patterns that have been passed down through your family. Considerable cleansing work may be needed to clear the imprints, memories and engrams from the past that are lodged here.

Karmic and ancestral issues: Memory, hereditary issues, sense perception.

Deeply ingrained soul programs, and emotional baggage from the past; the traumas, dramas, unfinished business, gifts and lessons learned over many lifetimes. This chakra may well be holding on to outdated soul intentions from previous lives.

Thought forms

Thought forms are created when people focus strongly upon something or have powerfully negative thoughts. In addition to being the product of your own mind, thought forms may arise from other people's perception or expectations, or from religious or other authoritarian dictates, and may also arise from books or films. Thought forms lodge themselves in the mental component of the subtle energy body as an internal thought form. Or, as external thought forms, inhabit the lower astral realms and attach to the chakras. External thought forms appear to have separate and distinct life and energy – and may interfere in the lives of human beings, typically by masquerading as a 'guide figure' who appears during meditation or quiet moments. Internal thought forms are usually experienced as a derogatory inner voice or obsessive thoughts. [See *Good Vibrations*]

The past life chakras link to 'junk DNA', genetic and cellular memory, the psoas muscle, the karmic blueprint and etheric bodies. Wounds, attitudes and dysfunction in these subtle bodies imprint on to the physical at a psychosomatic or genetic level. Psychological dis-eases impact on the mind and from there on to the body. Blockages here mean that you are stuck in the past and cannot move forward, and may well be repeating personal past life or ancestral patterns passed down through your family. Clearing the past life chakras means that you can move forward with no baggage, freed from the karmic energetic deficits or blockages that would prevent you from stepping into a new frequency. It also facilitates drawing on your karmic wisdom, the fruit of all your previous lives wherever they took place, and accessing ancestral wisdom.

To open the past life chakra
- *First ground yourself thoroughly (see page 19).*

- *Massage along the bony ridge at the back of the skull, working from just behind one ear and across to the other, with an appropriate crystal (see the Directory).*
- *Place the crystal in the central hollow at the top of the spine just below the ridge. If dizziness or nausea results, place an appropriate crystal on the soma chakra and breathe deeply into your grounding root until it subsides.*
- *Wait until the chakra stabilises before removing the crystals.*
- *If traumatic past life memories are triggered, use appropriate crystals and seek assistance from a qualified past life healer.*

To close the past life chakras

- *Slowly draw a Smoky Quartz, Flint, Hematite, Petrified Wood or other grounding crystal from behind one ear to the hollow at the base of the skull.*
- *Repeat for the other side.*
- *Place the crystal in the hollow and connect to the grounding cord.*

Third Eye/Brow

Location: Above and between the eyebrows.

Karmic level: Personal and ancestral.

The brow chakra is where your inner sight meets your outer sight and bonds into intuitive insight. It helps you to see beyond consensual reality into what really *is*. Imbalances here may create a sense of being bombarded by other people's thoughts, or irrational intuitions that have no basis in truth. Controlling or coercing mental 'hooks' from other people may lock in and affect your thoughts. An overactive brow creates a tendency to live in an escapist fantasy world, with a distorted view of reality. A blown chakra may replay dishonesty, evasiveness, impatience, pride, egotism or arrogance.

When too open, this chakra leaves you vulnerable to manipulation from those on other realms who may not have your highest good in mind. You may also act in a way that is manipulative and overbearing, feeling it is your god-given right. When the chakra is blocked, there may be unhealthy attachment to a belief system or a guru. Blockages often occur in this chakra, from childhood or other lives, especially if you have been discouraged from speaking about what you see – physically or metaphysically – or from following your own inner guidance. This quickly leads to self-doubt and a lack of trust in your intuition. When this occurs, there is a fear of success and 'imposter syndrome' (fear of being found out as not being who, or as capable as, you purport to be) is common.

Karmic issues: Metaphysical abilities, illusions and disillusions. Narrow-mindedness, fear and cynicism.

Soma

Location: Above the third eye, at the mid-hairline.

Karmic level: Soul, rejuvenation and immortality.

The soma is the anchor for the 'silver cord' that holds

the subtle energy bodies in contact with the physical. It has to do with perception of the cycles of time and awareness of the workings of synchronicity. When this chakra is functioning well, it gives you the mental clarity necessary to achieve en-lighten-ment. However, when this chakra is blown, it is all too easy for discarnate spirits to attach or for you to be subject to involuntary out-of-body experiences that may literally blow your mind.

Karmic and ancestral issues: Disconnection, dispossession, spiritual nourishment and connection.

Alta Major

Location: Inside the skull.

Karmic level: Karmic and ancestral.

The alta major gives the ability to see the bigger picture. All the pieces of the jigsaw puzzle of life fit in place. This chakra holds valuable information about the ancestral past and the ingrained patterns that govern human life and awareness. It, in conjunction with the causal vortex and past life chakras, contains your past life karma and the contractual agreements you made with your Higher Self and others before incarnating in this current lifetime. Activating it enables you to read your soul's plan. The alta major chakra governs the behavioural, autonomic, and endocrine functions that keep the body in harmony with external forces. It creates a direct pathway between your conscious, subconscious and intuitive minds and the higher universal mind.

When this chakra is blown memories flood in too fast

to process and overwhelm the psyche. Paradoxically, such memories of the past are clung to and govern behaviour. You may feel disorientated, open to paranoid delusions – which feel like reality – and are acutely attuned to subtle disturbances in the environment around you. You may feel like you've been taken over by something outside yourself. When this chakra is blocked, inner sight cannot open and new information cannot be processed. Transgenerational contracts and soul intention will be cut off from your conscious mind but may nevertheless affect your behaviour.

Karmic and ancestral issues: Control by the ancestors. Subtle dis-ease in all its forms.

To open the alta major

- *First ground yourself thoroughly (see page 19), placing an appropriate grounding crystal at your feet.*
- *Place an appropriate alta major crystal (see page 279) in the hollow at the base of the skull and one over the soma chakra. Blue or Black Moonstone at the base of the skull and Preseli Bluestone on the soma work well, as do Preseli Bluestone and Flint. If dizziness and nausea result, breathe deeply pushing the energy down into the grounding root. Wait until the chakra stabilises before removing the crystals.*

Note: This chakra very easily goes off balance and may need to be stabilised frequently during ancestral, karmic and soul healing as imprints and engrams are released and the vibrational frequency responds.

Crown

Location: Top of the head.

Karmic level: Personal, ancestral, collective and cosmic.

When the crown chakra connection is disturbed, you are disconnected from your spiritual self and from cosmic energies. Spiritual interference, or possession, may result and metabolic or psychological imbalances are common. If it is functioning well, you express yourself as a spiritual being and attain unity consciousness. Your soul purpose may be accessed and actualised, leading you to self-understanding. You will be certain of your pathway and in tune with the cycles of life. You will recognise the lessons you programmed in before birth and find the gift in their heart.

When this chakra is blown, it leads to an overly-imaginative, unfocused, spaced out and frustrated soul who is arrogant and uses power to control others. A blown crown is prey to illusions, undue influence and false communications. Obsession and openness to spiritual interference or possession may result. Attempting to control others is common, as is 'false guru' syndrome. Energy may rush back down to the sexual chakras causing a psychotic breakdown or obsessive sexual expression. When this chakra is blocked, it attracts put-downs and subtle attacks from others.

Karmic issues: Spiritual, intellectual and intuitive

knowing. Blocked sense of power, leading to egotism and alienation.

Causal Vortex ('Galactic')

Location: Above and behind the head to one side or the other (dowse for its exact placement).

Karmic level: Soul, cosmic and collective.

Acting rather like a universal and cosmic worlds wide web, the causal vortex is a conduit that accesses the Akashic Record especially that of your own soul and the ancestral line. It assists in assessing how far you have travelled on your spiritual journey and how well you are doing with your karmic lessons. When this chakra is operational, it receives wisdom and guidance from spiritual mentors and higher dimensional beings so that the soul's plan for the present lifetime may be amended when required. Accessing this chakra illuminates the things you have chosen to experience in a given physical life and what lessons you are trying to learn. It is also a repository for ancestral and karmic dis-eases. Cause and effect is understood dispassionately when viewed from the perspective of this chakra. There is no emotional involvement. When activated and developed, it keeps the connection to your soul open and helps you access your karmic skills and abilities. It keeps the mind clear and focused, allowing soul input, ideas and intuition to flow freely. This chakra can assimilate scalar wave energy, bringing the subtle and physical bodies into alignment and activating DNA potential that is carried in the consciousness between the cell walls. When the chakra is blocked or blown, you may be unconsciously propelled by your own past, ancestral or cultural imperatives or out of date soul contracts.

Karmic issues: Future and evolution of humanity. Your own karmic, ancestral or cultural imperatives.

To open the causal vortex

- *First ground yourself thoroughly. Place a grounding stone such as Flint or Smoky Quartz at your feet and picture a root going deep into the Earth (see page 19).*
- *Ascertain exactly where your causal vortex is as its location varies from person to person. It may be way out in your subtle energy field or fairly close to the skull. It is usually behind and to one side of the midline chakras. Dowse, sweep around your head with your palm chakra to sense its location, or use Blue Kyanite which 'sticks' or jumps when it reaches the chakra.*
- *Hold Blue Kyanite or other activation crystal over the chakra. If dizziness and nausea result, breathe deeply pushing the energy down into the grounding root. Placing an appropriate crystal such as Selenite, Flint or Preseli Bluestone on the soma chakra can also assist. Wait until the chakra stabilises before removing the crystals.*
- *When the chakra has stabilised, use the Kyanite crystal to gently draw its end nearer to the skull if it was far out in the energy field. This chakra is more like a tube than a flat disc and can be extended down from the*

Akashic Record into a more easily accessible layer of the etheric body.

To close the causal vortex

Hold Flint, Hematite, Petrified Wood or Smoky Quartz to create 'shutters' over the site.

Soul Star

Location: About a foot above your head.

Karmic level: Soul and collective.

An interface for relationship with the universe and beyond, the soul star is a bridge between spirit and matter. When not functioning at optimum, this chakra may lead to spiritual arrogance, soul fragmentation or a messiah complex. It is the person who rescues and enslaves others rather than empowering them. It may also be the site of spirit attachment, ET invasion, or overwhelm by ancestral spirits. When functioning at optimum there is true humility, with a connection to overall soul intention and an objective perspective on the past that leads to spiritual illumination. This chakra also holds the collective karma of humankind and the history of the evolution of the cosmos. When there is no control over this chakra it may lead to soul fragmentation or spirit attachment, ET invasion, or overwhelm by ancestral spirits and their unfulfilled desires.

If this chakra is blocked, there is little or no awareness of being an eternal spirit who happens to be in physical incarnation, and equally no connection to higher beings, or to your own higher energies. The viewpoint is consequentially narrow, materialistic and greedy or needy. You may well feel that you have no right to exist at all and constantly apologise for yourself. You may also feel that you are the cause of other people's problems and try to make reparation, or force a resolution on their behalf. Unresolved past life issues and previous soul imperatives may well be ruling your life.

Karmic issues: Unity consciousness, messiah complex, spiritual isolation, soul fragmentation.

Stellar Gateway

Location: Above the Soul Star.

Karmic level: Cosmic and soul.

The stellar gateway is a dimensional portal rather than a physical site. It is a point of connection to the divine and to the multiverses surrounding us: where the soul can make a connection to its own Higher Self, other realms, higher dimensions and All That Is. When this chakra is imbalanced the soul will be fragmented, disintegrated, unable to function in the everyday world. A blown stellar gateway leaves you open to illusions and to sources of cosmic disinformation. A blocked stellar gateway means you are unable to connect to your soul or higher dimensions. There is a feeling that the material realm is all that there is and so spiritual qualities such as empathy and compassion are lacking and ego runs rife.

Karmic and ancestral issues: Commitment to being incarnated on Earth, dispossession.

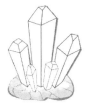

Opening the personal chakras and integrating the lesser known and higher vibration chakras

A simple crystal layout will cleanse and open the personal chakras so that the lesser known and higher vibration chakras can then be integrated into the system (see *Crystal Prescriptions volume 4*).

Personal chakra cleanse, balance and recharge

- *Place Smoky Quartz or other earth star crystal between and slightly below your feet. Picture light and energy radiating out from the crystal into the earth star for two or three minutes and be aware that the chakra is being cleansed and its spin regulated.*
- *Place Red Jasper or other base chakra crystal on the base chakra. Picture light and energy radiating out from the crystal into the base chakra as before.*
- *Place Orange Carnelian or other sacral chakra crystal on your sacral chakra, just below the navel. See the light and feel the cleansing process.*
- *Place Yellow Jasper or other solar plexus crystal on your*

solar plexus.

- *Place Green Aventurine or other heart chakra crystal on your heart.*
- *Place Blue Lace Agate or other throat chakra crystal on your throat.*
- *Place Sodalite or other third eye chakra crystal on your brow.*
- *Place Amethyst or other crown chakra crystal on your crown.*
- *Breathe deeply taking the breath all the way down to your feet as you inhale, and then letting your attention come slowly up your body as you exhale until you reach your crown. Repeat several times.*
- *Remain still and relaxed, breathing deep down into your belly and counting to seven before you exhale. As you breathe in and hold, feel the energy of the crystals re-energizing the chakras and from there radiating out through your whole being.*
- *Now take your attention slowly from the soles of your feet up the midline of your body feeling how each chakra has become balanced and harmonised.*
- *When you feel ready, gather your crystals up, starting from the crown. As you reach the earth star chakra, be aware of a grounding cord anchoring you to the Earth and into your physical body.*
- *Cleanse your stones thoroughly (see page 123).*

Alternatively: *Sweep Anandalite at arm's length from your feet up over your head and down to the floor behind you (you* *may need assistance to do this). If the crystal 'sticks', pause while it clears before moving on. Then sweep back up and over to the front again. Sweep side to side and back again as the chakras are like flat discs that extend in all directions.*

Integrating the lesser known chakras

Once the personal chakras are up and running efficiently, introduce the lesser known chakras such as the knees and the dantien into the above layout, placing an appropriate crystal. When the lesser known chakras have been cleansed and activated, allow the energy to flow and be incorporated into the personal chakra alignment. The higher chakras can then be incorporated into the layout. *See page 46 for past life chakra activation, page 53 for the causal vortex and page 50 for the alta major.*

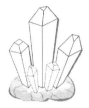

Higher chakra activation

This activation should be carried out with the basic chakras cleansed and open. Activate the chakras in order and do not rush the process. Open one at a time and give that chakra time to integrate into your entire chakra system before moving on to the next one. Allow yourself at least a week and probably longer to open and integrate all the higher chakras. Remember to open all the chakras up to the new chakra before beginning a fresh activation. You can dowse to check whether a higher chakra has already opened and come online, and when the opening and integration process is complete. This exercise is best done lying down as it facilitates placing the crystals and helps you to remain grounded.

Higher Chakra activation stages

- *Thoroughly ground yourself (see page 19).*
- *Complete the chakra rebalancing and recharging exercise.*
- *Then open the higher chakras slowly and in order, first placing a large Smoky Elestial, Hematite or other grounding stone below your feet to anchor the energies*

and a Selenite or Anandalite over your head.

- *Place a Gaia gateway chakra crystal on the Gaia gateway and feel it connect to the earth star to anchor all your energy bodies to the planet.*

- *Place a higher heart chakra crystal such as Rose Quartz, Danburite or Tugtupite over the higher heart chakra and leave it in place for two to five minutes. This chakra can be left open.*

- *Place a heart seed chakra crystal over the heart seed at the base of the breastbone and feel the influx of universal love that floods into the chakra and through your whole being. This chakra can be left open.*

- *When the higher heart and heart seed chakras have been opened, place crystals on all three heart chakras and feel the three-chambered heart chakra open and integrate. This chakra can be left open.*

- *Place a Preseli Bluestone or other cosmic anchor/soma chakra crystal such as Flint over the soma chakra. Open the chakra when you want to go journeying and close it when you want to stay in your physical body.*

- *Placing a high vibration crystal such as Selenite, Anandalite™ (Aurora Quartz), Rainbow Mayanite or Azeztulite on the soul star connects you to your soul and highest self. Invoke your Higher Self to guard it well. Be aware of its connection to the earth star. Close the chakra when not using the portal for journeying or guidance.*

- *Before opening the stellar gateway, invoke your guardian angel or other protective being to guard it well while you journey, meditate or seek guidance in other realms. Place Selenite, Anandalite, Phenacite, Rainbow Mayanite or other stellar gateway crystal to open the portal. Be aware of its connection to the Gaia gateway. Close the portal and the chakra when not in use.*

- *Use Anandalite™ (Aurora Quartz), Blue Kyanite, Blue Moonstone or other alta major chakra crystal to activate the alta major chakra. Place in the hollow at the base of the skull. Feel the Merkeba shape within your skull connect up all the systems within. If you feel at all lightheaded, take your attention down to the grounding stone at your feet and see page 19.*

- *To activate the causal vortex, see page 53.*

Remember to close each higher chakra when the activity is complete and open again before moving on to the next chakra activation. Close by visualising 'shutters' closing over them. Or, place a grounding crystal on the chakra.

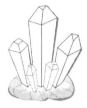

Chakra attachments

Chakras may be blocked by an attaching spirit, personal thought or belief, or imperatives or thought forms from the ancestral line. It's not only discarnate spirits that may attach here. The living may affect you too. It is quite common to find undue influence from the immediate family being exercised through the chakras – and through the navel if the influence is maternal. Thought is a very powerful thing and thought forms or strong belief systems may easily affect the chakras especially around the head and throat. It is also common to find that miscarriages or stillbirths have left behind some of the energy of the soul who could have been born, especially if there is an unfulfilled soul contract operating behind the scenes. You may find emotional attachment hooks in the spleen, sacral and solar plexus; thought forms in the third eye and soma; ancestral hooks operate in virtually all the chakras but especially the causal vortex, alta major, navel (tummy button) and base chakras.

Chakra attachments

Gaia Gateway (below the Earth Star): Planetary

connection

Attachments: Cosmic, racial and collective spirits, often those who were dispossessed of their lands or ethnically cleansed.

Earth Star (below the feet): Material connection

Attachments: Spirits of place, stuck spirits. Those who wish you to walk in their footsteps. If it is permanently open, you can easily pick up negative energies from the ground or attract 'spirits of place', either as attachments or as communication of events that have taken place.

Knee: Flexibility, balance and willpower

Attachments: Those who want you to walk in their footsteps – ancestral spirits or past life personas that have a different agenda to your present soul intentions.

Palm: Energy manifestation, transmutation and utilisation

Attachments: Energy drawn from anyone you've shaken hands with or touched in any way, also negative energy from objects or the environment. Anything you wished to hold on to in a previous life.

Base and sacral: Creativity

Attachments: Ancestral figures, previous partners, children, anyone you've ever had sex with, needy people, thought forms, unborn children and parents, disembodied sex addicts. Previous partners or significant others leave their imprint in these chakras and may continue to influence through the association. Sex addiction way back in the family may overstimulate these chakras and manifest in the present.

Dantien: Power

Attachments: Energy leeches, control freaks, disembodied spirits seeking energy to re-manifest or move on, past life personas, thought forms.

Navel: Nurturing

Attachments: The mother and the matriarchal line. Thought forms.

Solar plexus: Emotions

Attachments: People with whom you have had an emotional entanglement in the past whenever that may have been. Ancestral spirits, relatives, needy people. Invasion and energy leeching take place through this chakra. A 'stuck-open' solar plexus means you take on other people's feelings easily. You may well receive intuitions through your solar plexus as you unconsciously read other people's emotions.

Spleen (under left arm): Energy

Attachments: Psychic vampires, needy people, ex-partners, children. Psychic vampires can leech your energy and hooks here are common.

Heart seed (base of breastbone): Soul remembrance

Attachments: Parts of your soul left in other lives or dimensions. If you have left parts of yourself at past life deaths or traumatic or deeply emotional experiences, then these parts may be attached and trying to influence you to complete unfinished business.

Higher Heart (above the heart): Unconditional love

Attachments: Guides, gurus or masters, mentors. Not all masters or gurus have clean energy or the best of intentions.

Throat (over throat): Communication

Attachments: Teachers, mentors, gurus, thought forms. A blocked throat chakra results in difficulty in communication – especially in not being able to speak your truth. Problems may arise from your own unvoiced intuitions and the dogmatic nature of a blocked throat chakra may leave you closed to intuitive solutions.

Third Eye (slightly above and between the eyebrows): Intuition

Attachments: Thought forms, ancestors or relatives, lost souls. You may be attached to the past, fearful and superstitious, and prone to create exactly what you fear most.

Soma (above the third eye, at the hairline): Spiritual connection

Attachments: 'Lost souls', walk-ins, thought forms. When this chakra is stuck open, it is all too easy for spirits to attach.

Past life chakras (behind the ears along the bony ridge of the skull): Past experiences

Attachments: Past life personas, soul fragments, thought forms from previous beliefs. If the chakras are stuck open, you may feel unsafe and overwhelmed by past life memories of trauma and violent death and fears, which leaves the way open for past life personas and thought forms to attach or re-manifest.

Crown: Spiritual connection

Attachments: Spiritual entities, lost souls, mentors. If it is stuck open, then you may be prey to illusions and false communicators as it leaves you open to thought forms, spirit attachment or undue influence.

Soul Star (above your head): Spiritual enlightenment/ illumination

Attachments: Ancestral spirits, ETs, 'lost souls'. Stuck open or blocked, disturbances here may lead to soul fragmentation, spirit attachment, ET invasion, or overwhelm by ancestral spirits.

Stellar Gateway (above the Soul Star): Cosmic doorway to other worlds

Attachments: So-called enlightened beings that are

anything but. Delusion, deception and cosmic disinformation leaves you totally unable to function in the everyday world.

Causal Vortex (above and behind the head): The record of the soul's journey

Attachments: Past life and cultural or ancestral beliefs and soul imperatives, thought forms.

Alta Major (inside the head): Expanding awareness

Attachments: Memories from the past, thought forms carrying ancestral and karmic imperatives.

Releasing chakra attachments

Crystals can be used to 'clean out' hooks from the chakras. Flint, raw Charoite shards, Brandenberg, Lemurian Seed, Clear Quartz points and Stibnite work well. As does Rainbow Mayanite, particularly at a subtle level. Simply spiral the crystal in (counterclockwise is usual but use which works for you), then spiral the crystal out to pull out the attachments. Cleanse the crystal thoroughly and then spiral in light to seal where the attachment was held, or hold an Anandalite or other light bearing crystal over the site.

See *Crystal Prescriptions volume 4* for more detailed chakra work.

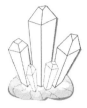

The aura and subtle energy bodies

The physical body is surrounded and interpenetrated by subtle energy fields or 'bodies' known as the aura or biomagnetic sheath. The aura is linked through, but not limited to, specific chakras. All, or any, of the subtle bodies may hold personal karmic or ancestral trauma, engrams and imprints that need to be released and healed. These subtle energy bodies with their imprints radiate out from the body in layers, with the chakras connecting them, each having a finer and more subtle vibration. But they are actually interlinked through multidimensional frequencies and interpenetrate each other. Crystals interact with the chakras and the blueprints to bring the bodies back into an appropriate harmony and equilibrium and to heal energetic 'holes', energy loss, distortion or imprinted patterns that no longer serve you.

Aura

The subtle biomagnetic sheath around the physical body that holds the energetic imprint of your present and former lives, and those of the ancestors.

These interpenetrating layers are like blueprints that hold information, bio-memories and engrams from which the physical body will be constructed and maintained. The blueprints affect how the chakras function as well as your physical, emotional and mental well-being. In some cases, blockages in the chakras may need to be released by healing the subtle energy body first. In other cases, clearing the chakra will result in clearing a specific layer of the subtle energy body. Medical science is beginning to recognise the existence of these bio-memory blueprints.

Bio-memories are memories that are locked into our cells. They carry hereditary memories, past-life memories and memories that have become part of the very fiber of our current personality through constant repetition for years. Both physical and mental patterns can become part of our bio-memory. Bio-memories have the power to trigger physical actions like fight or flight. Mental states like depression and anxiety can quickly become part of our bio-memory if we are not careful. Bio-memories are not only unconscious, but are usually untraceable to any particular source incident.[3]

These bio-memories are also known as engrams, or engraved memories, and are:

bio-chemical changes that occur in neural tissues as the result of a powerful or persistent reaction to any situation. An engram is not an ordinary memory, but more like a photograph of the situation or event, complete with the emotional response that accompanied it. Engrams exist just below the level of our consciousness, influencing our emotional responses without our knowledge.

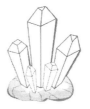

The Subtle Bodies

Physical etheric body

The physical subtle body, or etheric blueprint, tends to be closest in vibration to the physical body and can often be seen with a psychic eye as a white aura around that body. It is a biomagnetic program and holds imprints of past life dis-ease, injuries and beliefs, which present life symptoms then replay. It also holds subtle DNA that may be activated, or switched off, by behaviour and beliefs, and which in turn affects DNA in the physical body. It is connected through the seven traditional, lower frequency chakras on the body, and the soma, past life, alta major and causal vortex.

Emotional etheric body

The emotional body is created by emotions and feelings, attitudes, heartbreaks, traumas and dramas, not only in the present life but in previous lives. Emotional dis-ease shows up as dark or distorted patches within the subtle emotional body, the solar plexus and heart chakras. The emotional body may contain engrams, bundles of energy that hold a deeply traumatic or joyful memory picture.

Dis-ease in this body may also be reflected in the sacral and base chakras, and the knees and feet which will act out insecurities and fears.

Mental etheric body

The mental body is created by thoughts, memories, credos and ingrained beliefs from both the present and previous lives. It is connected particularly strongly through the throat and head chakras, but may be reflected in the lower body chakras also. This body holds the imprint of all that has been said or taught by authority figures in the past along with inculcated ideologies and points of view. It may need to be cleared and reprogrammed with a perspective more suitable to the current stage of spiritual growth so that it opens the way for evolution on all levels.

Karmic etheric body

The karmic body or blueprint holds the imprint of all previous lives and the purpose for the present life. This means that it contains mental programs, physical imprints, and emotional impressions and beliefs that you hold about yourself, many of which may be contradictory as they may arise from very different experiences in various lives. When the karmic body is healed, evolutionary intent may be actualised. This body is accessed through the past life, alta major and causal vortex chakras but may also affect the soma, knee and earth star.

Ancestral etheric body

The ancestral body holds all that you have inherited down your ancestral lines on both sides, everything your ancestors passed on to you either at the physical or more subtle levels. This may include family sagas, belief systems and attitudes, culture and expectations, traumas and dramas that shape your world. Healing sent back down the ancestral line to the core experience rebounds forward to heal the line going out into the future, making change possible. This body can be accessed through the soul star, past life, alta major, higher heart, earth star and Gaia gateway chakras. It has a great deal to do with how much at home you feel on the planet and whether you are able to put your soul purpose into practice. You may need to release ancestral expectations from this body before soul evolution can occur.

Planetary etheric body

While you are in incarnation, you also have a subtle energy body that links into the planet and the Earth's etheric body and meridians. This planetary body is connected to the wider cosmos, the luminaries, planets and stellar bodies and the outer reaches of the universe. Through this planetary body you are, therefore, connected into the wider whole. The planetary body is reflected in your birthchart and is accessed through the past life, alta major, causal vortex, soma, stellar and Gaia gateway chakras. Cosmic or soul dis-ease can be corrected through the planetary subtle body in addition to ancestral and genealogical karma.

Spiritual body or Lightbody

The spiritual body or lightbody is an integrated, luminous, vibrating energy field consisting of the physical body and all the subtle energy bodies, plus the spirit or soul, connected through all the chakras but especially through the higher dimensional ones: soma, soul star, stellar gateway, Gaia gateway, alta major and causal vortex. It is an electromagnetic field of varying oscillation with integrated frequencies from the highest to the lowest: being light in all its varied manifestations. The body itself resonates with the universe, the universal mind and with your own soul or spirit. When the lightbody is activated, it can literally re-encode your 'junk DNA' bringing out its highest potential and allowing your soul's purpose to manifest.

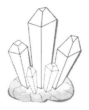

To harmonise the subtle energy bodies and integrate the chakras

Harmonising and integrating the chakras and auric bodies before you begin work on karmic or ancestral healing assists the process.

- *Hold a piece of Anandalite or other subtle body harmoniser in your hand and sweep it at arm's length from your feet up over your head and down to your feet at the back – if you find it difficult to reach ask a friend to assist. Then bring it up and over your head again and back to the floor.*
- *Sweep it from one side of your body to the other moving from your feet up over your head and down to your feet on the other side. Return to the first side.*
- *You may have to carry out several sweeps moving your arm closer in each time to integrate and harmonise all the subtle bodies with the higher dimensional energetic levels of the chakras.*
- *Place a piece of Flint at your feet and repeat the grounding exercise on page 19.*

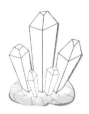

The psoas, 'soul muscle', and the bodymind

By learning to relax my psoas I was literally energizing my deepest core by reconnecting with the powerful energy of the earth... the psoas is far more than a core stabilizing muscle; it is an organ of perception composed of bio-intelligent tissue and "literally embodies our deepest urge for survival, and more profoundly, our elemental desire to flourish."

Danielle Prohom Olson,
www.bodydivineyoga.wordpress.com

The psoas muscle is the core-stabilising muscle of the body, connecting as it does the torso and the legs. It is the major muscle for keeping you upright and moving forward. In addition to connecting the legs and spine, the psoas is energetically attached to the diaphragm and so affects breathing. When the psoas muscle is tense, and especially when it is holding traumatic patterns, it affects your structural balance and your ability to stay in the present moment. It can hold deep seated anxiety and fear, keeping the physical body in permanent 'fight or flight' mode. In the Taoist tradition, the psoas is known as 'the muscle of the soul'. It holds both soul and ancestral memories within it. This muscle surrounds the lower dantien: a major energy centre of body sited just below the navel. The dantien is where you store your life force and your power, and which is the centre of gravity for your body. Release psoas tension and it can have a dramatic effect on the body in just a few minutes – although nausea, muscle spasm and trembling thighs might accompany the initial release. Peace of mind is restored, allowing the life force energy to flow freely around the body once more. A flexible and strong psoas also grounds you on to the planet, acting like an earthing wire.

Is your psoas contracted?

- *Do you feel pulled off balance?*
- *Is your lower body twisted away from your upper torso?*
- *Does it feel like you are permanently 'walking against the wind'?*
- *Do you feel like you're on a boat rather than on solid ground?*
- *Do you suffer from permanent headaches, nausea, vertigo, back or knee pain?*
- *Is there a discrepancy in the position of your knees?*

Relaxing the psoas and releasing the past

This exercise utilises your bodymind memory and releases tightness and patterns held in the psoas muscle, lessening the fight or flight response and calming anxiety. It is important that you do not judge the feelings you find within yourself. Simply acknowledge and accept them. Set aside at least half an hour for the exercise and be sure to turn off your mobile phone. It will become quicker the more you work with it. It is helpful to have a friend assist with this exercise at first to place the crystals when appropriate, and also find additional crystals that you may need. If you are working alone, before you begin, place your crystals where you will be able to reach them easily.

You will need:

- A heart seed chakra crystal (see the Directory, page 328)
- Magnesite or other muscle releasing crystal (see the Directory, page 344)
- Two Ancestralite or other deep programming release crystals (see PTSD, releasing fear or flash-backs entries in the Directory)
- Flint, Smoky Quartz or other grounding crystal
- A heart healing crystal such as Danburite, Mangano Calcite
- Selenite or Anandalite
- Brandenberg Amethyst
- Any other crystal for an identified fear or emotion

A drummed heartbeat rhythm assists this exercise.

Exercise: Healing the psoas muscle

- *Lie down in the foetal position: legs curled up, head down on your chest, arms wrapped around yourself.*
- *Take four or five deep, slow breaths, breathing right down into your belly and pausing between each in and out breath.*
- *Use your mind to scan your body and your feelings. Do not judge what you find. If there is a pain or tightness, simply acknowledge it. If there is a feeling or deep emotion, acknowledge the feeling, allow it to be there, and notice where it lives in your body. Do not judge it as 'good' or 'bad'. Simply accept it. Continue to breathe rhythmically as you do so.*
- *After five minutes or so, slowly open your arms, straighten your legs, raise your head and turn on to your back with your arms open and out to the side. Again, notice how you feel, but do not judge. Simply acknowledge and allow.*
- *Move your arms loosely by your side, elbows bent out and palms turned upwards.*
- *Now bend your legs up.*
- *Gently flex your lower back. Raising it up off the floor an inch or so and then allowing it to relax and flatten again.*
- *Straighten your right leg and slowly lower it to the floor. If you can raise your leg and straighten it in the air without discomfort before lowering it, do so. If not slide your foot along the floor. Relax the knee so that the leg is as flat as possible (a cushion under your knees*

may make you more comfortable).

- *Flex your lower back up again and then flatten it.*
- *Breathe.*
- *Flex your back once again and then slowly lower your left leg.*
- *Flex your back again and breathe.*
- *Your legs should be slightly parted and in a comfortable position, knees relaxed, feet flopping wherever they feel comfortable.*
- *Place a Smoky Quartz or other grounding stone at your feet (sit up to do this if you are working alone).*
- *Place a heart seed chakra stone at the base of your breastbone and a muscle releasing crystal underneath under your back about a hand's breadth above your waist.*
- *If you became aware of a strong emotion or feeling or pain or tightness while you were in the foetal position, you can position an appropriate crystal over the site.*
- *Place Anandalite, Selenite or other appropriate light-bringing crystal above your head taking your arms as far up as they'll go.*
- *Hold an Ancestralite or other crystal in your hands and lay them in your groin crease on either side.*
- *Ask your friend to loosely cover you with a light blanket to keep you warm. Lie still for at least five or ten minutes, preferably fifteen (the time can lengthen with practice). If you become uncomfortable, bring your legs up again and perform the back flexes and legs stretches while keeping keep the Ancestralite or other crystal in*

your groin creases. (If it becomes uncomfortable, place a cushion under your knees to support them.)

- Be aware of the light flooding down through you from the Anandalite or other crystal above your head and the crystal at your feet drawing off discomfort and toxicity and replacing it with light.
- When you feel thoroughly detoxified, add the Brandenberg crystal just above the heart seed crystal or on your forehead, whichever feels most comfortable. Spend five minutes or so in this position simply allowing the crystal to amend your energetic blueprint.
- Sharp twitches, or energetic releases, are quite common during this process, as is trembling of your thighs. Simply breathe gently and easily and allow them to happen.
- If you have appropriate dramatic drum or gong music, you can play this during the latter part of the process.
- If you became aware of a particularly strong emotion or feeling during the foetal position stage or at any other time, allow yourself to stay a little longer and play appropriate gong or drumming music whilst holding pieces of Ancestralite in your groin crease. Other crystals or shells that hold deep music within them may be appropriate to place around you. Go with the flow, which may well sound like a wave or moving water. When the feeling has been released, do the back flexes and leg stretches to loosen and release the psoas muscle and return to lie on your back. Place your Brandenberg wherever it feels appropriate and allow it to input the

perfect pattern in to your energy field. As each person is
unique, you will need to follow your intuition on this.

The psoas muscle anchor

A simpler, but nevertheless equally profound, release is
found in the psoas muscle anchor. Once again, do not
judge any feelings that arise, simply allow them to
intensify and then dissipate naturally as the muscle
lengthens and releases.

- *Place a Smoky Quartz or other grounding stone point down at your feet, point down.*
- *Place a Flint or other grounding stone at the base of the breastbone, point down.*
- *Place Charoite or other knee chakra stones on the knees. Feel your knees relax.*
- *Place a Magnetite or other muscle relaxing stone in the groin crease on each side.*
- *Place Rose Quartz over the heart chakra (just above the Smoky Quartz).*
- *Place your hands over the crystals in your groin creases.*
- *Lie quietly, breathing deep into the base of your belly for five minutes.*

This layout also works very well using Celtic or Clear
Quartz on all the points.

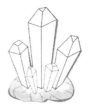

Breaking the code: 'junk DNA'

In the movie Superman, *the infant Kal-El is sent in a crystal capsule to Earth, with ethereal sounds and images to teach him along the way. The crystals were then stored in a crystal cave for his future use. All knowledge was imbedded in the crystals. How true this is! All the healing knowledge we humans need to access and know about has been imbedded and stored in the crystals of our own DNA. Crystals can transmit information to us, about survival, about our past and about healing. We just need to access, to listen, and be open to the possibilities.*

Kathy M. Scogna, foreword to Junk DNA: Unlocking the Hidden Secrets of Your DNA

Personal trauma and transgenerational memories are also held in so-called 'junk DNA', affecting the karmic blueprint and our subtle energy fields. The karmic blueprint carries the impact of all our experiences from life to life *in whatever dimension that they may have occurred*. 'Junk DNA', the subtle blueprints and the Akashic Record are part of our inner landscape. In addition to our own personal stuff, 'junk DNA' is what gets passed down through the ancestral line so it's where we tune in to a vast field of experience much wider than our own. It is found in each cell of our bodies, so it has important implications for who you are, on many levels. Crystals such as Brandenberg Amethyst, Cradle of Life (Humankind), Lakelandite and Ancestralite assist the healing and transformation process for these fields and the remedy flawed 'junk DNA'. Brandenberg holds the perfect blueprint before anything was imprinted and can, therefore, return the energy to a state of perfection. But Ancestralite takes this a step further and carries forward the soul learning, while at the same time healing the ancestral wounds and so assists soul evolution.

But what exactly is 'junk DNA'?

Well, briefly it's what the genetic scientists couldn't immediately identify the purpose of when unravelling the secrets of DNA. It didn't 'code'. So they called it 'junk' and relegated it to the dustbin. All 98% of it. Maybe it's time to think more in terms of a recycling opportunity. Because one thing is now certain, junk it is not. Genie might be a more appropriate expression:

Junk. Barren. Non-functioning. Dark matter. *That's how scientists had described the 98% of human genome that lies between our 21,000 genes, ever since our DNA was first* sequenced *about a decade ago. The disappointment in those descriptors was intentional and palpable. It had been believed that the human genome – the underpinnings of the blueprint for the talking, empire-building, socially evolved species that we are – would be stuffed with sophisticated genes, coding for critical proteins of unparalleled complexity. But when all was said and done, and the Human Genome Project finally determined the entire sequence of our DNA in 2001, researchers found that the 3 billion base pairs that comprised our mere 21,000 genes made up a paltry 2% of the entire genome. The rest, geneticists acknowledged with unconcealed embarrassment, was an apparent biological wasteland. But it turns out they were wrong. In an impressive series of more than 30 papers published in several journals,* including Nature, Genome Research, Genome Biology, Science *and* Cell, *scientists now report that these vast stretches of seeming 'junk' DNA are actually the seat of crucial gene-controlling activity.*[4]

Many researchers are in fact exploring the pseudogenome of humans or other organisms as a sort of molecular paleontology to better understand evolutionary history... [online forum][5]

If I'm interpreting a comment from an online forum correctly, it sounds like it's confirming that 'junk DNA' carries soul or ancestral memory. And, what is even more exciting, it indicates that the 'junk DNA' can indeed be changed and used for healing the past:

Pseudogenes are also important for ongoing evolution.

Because many of them still have gene promoters, valid open reading frames, and stop codons, but are not required for the organism's survival or development, they can function sort of like evolutionary sandboxes. Starting from a functional gene, mutations are freely introduced that could lead to radical changes in protein function. It's been found again and again that pseudogenes actually do get expressed sometimes when an organism is stressed, so if beneficial mutations have been introduced, they may help the organism survive and might be more permanently up-regulated in the offspring.[6]

Jumping genes or should that be genies?

This opens up new possibilities for switching off inappropriate and detrimental genetic responses and switching on positive, beneficial effects:

Transposable elements (TEs), also known as 'jumping genes' or transposons, are sequences of DNA that move (or jump) from one location in the genome to another. Maize geneticist Barbara McClintock discovered TEs in the 1940s, and for decades thereafter, most scientists dismissed transposons as useless or 'junk' DNA. McClintock, however, was among the first researchers to suggest that these mysterious mobile elements of the genome might play some kind of regulatory role, determining which genes are turned on and when this activation takes place (McClintock, 1965).

DNA affects psychological and physiological processes.

The actions of the DNA and RNA are necessary to put the whole system into operation. The specific fluids that surround the DNA are in precise quantities, which can be translated by a crystalline mirror-like structure, like a laser beam, throughout the entire system. Thus the passages of processes, whether these are electrical, electrochemical or purely chemical, can follow a precise mirrored blueprint.[7]

If we can turn our genetic memory on or off, making use of those 'jumping genes', it has enormous implications for our health, well-being – and evolution. It's been shown that traumas, dramas and indeed belief systems can affect our DNA. Kathy Scogna's late husband, Joe, likened our DNA to a computer memory chip with RAM – Random Access Memory: something we can all access – and change.

The DNA that Joe embraced and wrote about was not just the physical DNA but rather the holistic DNA, the body, mind and spirit DNA of all life energy forms, all of this stored in our very own RAM chip. When understood in this context, the entire composition and view of DNA changes. We see the inherited personality traits, our own emotional traumas and the emotional upsets and behaviour of our parents being acted out in the genetic plans and blueprints we have been bequeathed from ages past to understand and process. Yes, our DNA can be changed and altered in so many ways, by our own environment and our adventures and misadventures in life.[8]

Kathy Scogna summarises the formation of our DNA as follows:

> *What has occurred on earth from the beginning of time with its geological transformations and eras, with its progression of creatures and energies needing protection, all this has been left as tracings within our DNA. The gravitational, radiational and magnetic flows in the solar system, the beginning of life in the seas and on land with those biological tracings, and the sounds, utterances (languages) and the history of our species has been recorded as well.*
>
> *We are products of our ancestors on a cellular level, going back even earlier than Stone Age man with all the beliefs, traumas and behaviours intact and products of our environment (learning, people, places and events), as well as being products of what we eat, breathe in and drink, all to be discovered and rectified, when necessary, by intense mental and spiritual conditioning. This work embraces both creation and evolution…*

Crystals too are a product of their environment and the processes through which they have evolved. To my mind, they hold the purest energy pattern: one that is radiated to us through their vibrations. That's why they can bring us back into balance – and help us to evolve. Kathy Scogna again:

> *What is the language of DNA in the crystalline structures*

that acts much like a laser beam? The vibration of sonic waves. Frequencies. This is a multi-way communication line, in and out, so that we have input as well: words read, spoken or sung, thoughts, emotions and other 'emotional radiation', as well as telepathic messages from a distance are involved in the process.

Scalar waves

Everything is energy and that everything vibrates at different frequencies. Bio-scalar energy is a unique form of energy that can be harnessed and directed into solid objects or bodies placed in its field.

Kalon Prensky

Scalar waves are found throughout the universe and within our physical bodies. Bioscalar wave energy exists at the microscopic level in the nucleus of an atom or a cell and creates a bioenergetic source more powerful than DNA, cellular matrixes and other physiological processes. Whilst some bioscalar waves may be viewed as harmful, beneficial bioscalar waves have been shown to energize the extracellular matrix of the body and protect against electromagnetic emanations and geopathic stress that would otherwise detrimentally affect cells and tissue. They activate the meridians and facilitate healing at the energetic interface between spirit and matter.[9] It is probable that all healing crystals have this energy within their matrix, and that their crystalline structure actually produces bioscalar energy. If, as Lilli

Botchis asserts, "when the human body enters a scalar wave field, the electromagnetic field of the individual becomes excited [and] this catalyzes the mind/body complex to return to a more optimal state that is representative of its original, natural, electrical matrix form,"[10] we can see how a crystal with its optimal energy pattern might operate on the human and planetary energy body... The "active spinning vortices composed of quantities of energy that interact with all non-physical dimensions including consciousness" can be anywhere and everywhere instantaneously and simultaneously. Like two piano strings with the same tone, energy can be exchanged and aligned through resonance and vibration. Many if not all crystals generate scalar waves... A quick look at current definitions of scalar waves shows us that they are intelligent and proactive and indicates how they might function in crystal healing:

A scalar wave is non-linear, *not electromagnetic, and exists in multiple dimensions beyond time or space. That means they do not decay with time or distance from their source. Scalar waves can interact with all matter including electromagnetism but since they are non-linear and hyperspatial, they... must be detected and measured indirectly... A scalar transmitter can wirelessly send power to a receiver through any obstacle... [even] a Faraday Cage or a metal box, and a receiver can receive power far away. During the process of transmission and reception they can magnify power. (www.homeotronics.com)*

A Scalar Wave is not a single wave but a result of the inter-action (interference) of multiple waves of very high frequency which seem to modulate and encode each other in a harmonious holistic complexity, similar to a hologram. The resulting multidimensional standing wave pattern emanates out of a fixed source point (a healer) [or crystal] and can be received and decoded by a similar resonant quantum-connected receiver point (recipient)... This causes vibrational ripples in the Morphogenic Field of the Cosmic Unified Field. (www.keylonticdictionary.org)
[Extracted from *Crystal Prescriptions volume 3*]

So. Link scalar waves and crystals with 'junk DNA' and you have a mechanism for evolutionary and ancestral change.

Healing 'junk DNA'

Positive affirmations, EFT and the like work, all work, by interacting with the random access memory of our DNA and unlocking its hold – especially through the magical jumping genie of our 'junk' DNA. A process that I find is facilitated and eased by holding a crystal. One of the latest ones to come my way is the Cradle of Life (Humankind), an extraordinary healer for ancestral, personal and planetary DNA. Try gridding it around you in whatever pattern comes to you intuitively and let the genies jump out of the bottle to transform you! Many of the exercises in this book also transform your 'junk' DNA, releasing its potential.

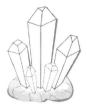

Post-traumatic stress disorder

The effect of PTSD can be far-reaching. PTSD can be a debilitating disorder, and its symptoms can have a negative impact on a number of different areas in a person's life. In particular, PTSD can negatively affect a person's mental health, physical health, work, and relationships… But in the midst of such grim findings, scientists also sound a note of hope for PTSD patients and their loved ones. According to them, by delving into the pathophysiology of PTSD, they have also realized that the disorder is reversible. The human brain can be re-wired… The brain is a finely-tuned instrument. It is fragile, but it is heartening to know that the brain also has an amazing capacity to regenerate. [http://healthwatchwi.com/tag/ptsd/]

PTSD is a graphic reliving of previous trauma through vivid flashbacks and nightmares. I am including the subject of post-traumatic stress disorder (PTSD) in this section because it can have ancestral (transgenerational), soul and karmic aspects as well as personal present life experiences. They play out in the background at varying levels and in different ways according to the area of life where the PTSD first arose – which may be many lifetimes 'back in time' although in fact in PTSD there is no time as such. The trauma remains in the now. In transgenerational stress passed down a family, the person experiencing the subtle symptoms of PTSD may have no knowledge of its source. Some, but not all, memories of personal past lives may in fact be genetically transmitted ancestral memories. Although it is not uncommon for a soul to reincarnate into the same, or a similar, family line in order to heal the effects of the original trigger event.

It is not only the human brain that can regenerate in such situations; the human soul is indestructible no matter how battered or intermittently fragmented it may become. This is where the major healing needs to occur (see Part III). The effects of which are then transmitted to the physical level of being. However, the original stressor event may create thought forms that will need to be dissolved (see page 255) and soul retrieval may well be necessary (page 204) in addition to returning any spirit attachments to the light (see page 214). Healing PTSD in the present moment not only heals the past but also transmutes it so that is not transmitted to future generations.

Symptoms of PTSD

- Intrusive recollections – vivid flashbacks and nightmares
- Inability to recall trigger event
- Fragmented soul
- Chronic fatigue

- Hyperarousal: constantly on high alert – 'flight or fight' mode permanently switched on
- Suppressed cortisol levels
- Dissociation ('checking out')
- Functioning on 'automatic pilot'
- 'Memory out of whack', unreliable, confused and intermittent
- False memory syndrome
- Inability to correctly interpret an environmental context – emotions and physical reactions occur in the body that do not relate to what is going on in the moment
- Inability to control emotional responses
- Emotional anaesthesia – 'numbness'
- Toxic emotions – shame, fear, anger, guilt, agitation
- Extreme emotional reactions
- Inability to experience positive emotions or enjoy activities – life is 'flat, lacklustre and depressed'
- Excessive 'startle response'
- Paranoia, feeling unsafe. Tendency to be jumpy and uncomfortable around people.
- Panic attacks
- Self-destructive activities
- Addiction to danger, drugs, alcohol
- Constant, extreme stress levels
- Insomnia
- Suicidal feelings
- Head or stomach aches, bowel problems
- 'Frozen in time' – suspended in the past

- Avoidance of people, places, activities or thoughts that reactivate memories
- Negative belief system, e.g. 'the world is a bad place'

[Extracted from http://healthwatchwi.com/tag/ptsd/ with additions by Judy Hall]

> **Flashback:** A spontaneous remembering of a past life or traumatic event. It may come out of the blue or be triggered by a place (déjà vu), person or object, or by touching the part of the body involved in the memory. All the senses will be involved: sight, sound, touch and smell.

PTSD and previous lives

PTSD does not simply occur from present life experiences. Previous life, intrauterine experience, and ancestral trauma may also create PTSD *as may living on the site of an old trauma in those who are psychically sensitive.*

Stressors that trigger re-emergence

- Event or emotional challenge which mirrors original cause
- Major life event
- Change in relationship(s)
- Lack of social support

- Lack of validation
- Vulnerability from previous trauma reignited by current events
- Interpersonal violation – especially by trusted others
- Actual or symbolic loss
- Beliefs are challenged by events
- Shattering of illusions and defensive walls
- Return to the site or source
- Regression techniques
- Touching a vulnerable part of the body

The hippocampus

Grid cells have attracted attention because the crystal-like structure underlying their firing fields is not, like in sensory systems, imported from the outside world, but is created within the brain itself… the map is associated with specific features and experiences, forming individualized maps that are stored in the neural networks of this brain region.
May-Britt Moser and Edvard I. Moser[11]

The hippocampus is where new brain cells are born and where memories are mediated.[12] It actually contains natural Magnetite crystals within it.[13] According to Health Watch, "The most significant neurological impact of trauma is seen in the hippocampus. PTSD patients show a considerable reduction in the volume of the hippocampus. This region of the brain is responsible for memory functions. It helps an individual to record new memories and retrieve them later in response to specific and relevant environmental stimuli. The hippocampus, a direction finder 'compass', also helps us distinguish between past and present memories."

This means that PTSD patients no longer have the ability to discriminate between past and present. As a result, minor stressors that have very little to do with the initial trigger may have a profound impact, recreating an event as though it is happening in the present moment. Health Watch use the example of a rape victim for whom any car park will trigger a reliving because the first event occurred around parked cars. However, the fact that there are crystalline structures within the hippocampus means that crystals can be used to entrain the hippocampus back to more appropriate functioning. Preseli Bluestone or Fluorapatite is particularly useful in resetting the hippocampus, but see the A–Z Directory. And the even better news is that, as the hippocampus is where new brain cells are born, neuroplasticity means that fresh cells can forge new pathways and new memories, a process enhanced by meditation, relaxation and crystal entrainment.

> *By using our mind (spirit/will) to calm ourselves the new cells born in the hippocampus can help the brain forge new pathways [through] neuroplasticity.*
> Dan Siegel, "Understanding how your mind can heal your brain."

Neuroplasticity: "The brain's ability to reorganize itself by forming new neural connections throughout life. Neuroplasticity allows the neurons (nerve cells) in the brain to compensate for injury and disease and to adjust their activities in response to new situations or to changes in their environment."
http://www.medicinenet.com

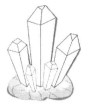

PTSD healing layout

This layout calls back, heals and integrates any parts of the soul that have been left at the point of trauma, soothes the heart and reconnects to a purer 'divine' source energy rather than old, bruised personal or ancestral energy. It sends healing down the ancestral line if required. For this layout, find yourself a quiet place where you will not be disturbed. Switch off your phone and lie down comfortably. Ensure you are warm enough and that there will be no loud noises to break into your silence. If you find it difficult to remain still and silent, a shamanic drumming track played quietly in the background may be helpful as it will entrain your heartbeat and brainwaves into relaxation mode.

- *Place a grounding stone at your feet and put your grounding cord in place (see page 19).*
- *Place Blue Kyanite or other healing crystal on the causal vortex chakra above your head (dowse for its placement in advance if necessary as it may be located above or to one side or other of your head, see page 53).*
- *Place Nuummite, Preseli Bluestone or other healing*

crystal on the forehead.

- *Place Kunzite, Danburite or other healing crystal on the heart.*
- *Place Black Tourmaline or other detoxifying crystal on the base chakra.*
  - *If there is a past life or transgenerational component to the PTSD, placing Ancestralite or other appropriate ancestral or karmic healing stone in the hollow at the base of the neck or held in your hands over your sacral chakra is helpful.*
  - *If there is an abuse or assault component, several Mangano Calcite, Rose Quartz or other abuse-healing crystals placed around the navel and close to the heart is helpful. A Shiva Lingam or Shiva Shell between the base and sacral chakra may also assist.*
- *Breathe gently and slowly, establishing a regular pattern. Pause between breaths and make the out breath longer than the in.*
- *Repeat quietly to yourself: "I am safe, I am healed, I am protected. I forgive and let go." (If there is a transgenerational component add: "We are safe, we are healed, we are protected. We all forgive and let go.")*
- *Leave stones in place for 15–20 minutes.*
- *Carry one of the stones with you at all times and repeat the affirmation if a stressor trigger occurs.*

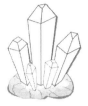

Breaking the PTSD response and stuck memory syndrome – EMDR

EMDR (Eye Movement Desensitization and Reprocessing) is one of the 'first aid' methods used in the field and as a treatment therapy by health professionals to desensitise 'stuck memory' syndrome. It is equally useful for treating past life memories, phobias or trans-generational trauma. EMDR uses rapid eye movements to shift focus and take you into a calm space. Using a crystal with distinctive markings can assist your eyes to make the movements. Choose a flat faced, chunky crystal with pronounced bands or spirals (Shiva Shells, Banded Agate, Black Sardonyx and Malachite are excellent) and keep it in your pocket ready for action. This exercise works particularly well if you have the picture or feeling of the trauma in your mind, but it will also work if you concentrate on the feeling that a trigger has aroused in you. Do not try to push either the picture or the feeling away; instead let it fade naturally as your eyes move around the crystal.

Breaking the response

- *When a memory or feeling surfaces, hold the crystal level with your eyes with your arm partially bent. Have the crystal as close to you as possible so that it fills your field of vision.*
- *Look left and focus on the topmost corner at the starting point of a band.*

> *If using a circular banded crystal, follow the circle right around to your starting point i.e. move your eyes clockwise as you are facing it.*
>
> *If using a spiral crystal, follow the spiral into the centre and out again.*
>
> *If using a straight-banded crystal, look left. Lift your eyes up to the topmost corner of the crystal and move across looking left to right. Drop your gaze down to the bottom corner and then back towards your starting point on your left. When you reach the left, lift your eyes up to your starting point at the top.*

- *Time your breathing to fit in with the movements:*
  - *Breathe in as you go across to the right.*
  - *Breathe out as you go down and back to the left.*
  - *Begin to breathe in again as you move up to your starting point.*
  - *Repeat the cycle.*
- *As you do so, repeat to yourself, "This is a just a memory, it is fading, I am healing."*
  - *If you are using a Shiva Shell, follow the line into the centre and then reverse direction and out again ten–twenty times.*

○ *If you are using Banded Agate or Malachite, follow the lines around in one direction for seven circles and then reverse direction for seven circles.*

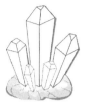

Crystal EFT

EFT (the Emotional Freedom Technique) may be used to clear both your own karmic and internal issues and those of the ancestors. The technique involves 'tapping' a series of points on the body and you can use your own body as a surrogate. Use of a crystal such as a Brandenberg or other Quartz point dramatically increases the transformation process as the crystal absorbs and transmutes the energy released during the tapping. Points are tapped with the flat or rounded end rather than sharp point of the crystal to avoid possibility of injury. If a point needs to be tapped using all the fingers, hold the crystal in the palm of your hand with your thumb. Remember to cleanse the crystal thoroughly after each use and, if it feels necessary, between each round of tapping.

You may need several sessions of tapping to reverse the deepest cause of issues, especially if you are working on behalf of the ancestral line or clearing transgenerational trauma. When tapping, simply follow your instincts and allow yourself to say anything that comes to mind no matter how ludicrous or unlikely it may sound. This free-flow, stream of consciousness combined with loving compassion and forgiving acceptance of yourself or the ancestors uncovers, releases and transforms the issues. It puts you in touch with toxic thoughts and buried emotions that unknowingly lurk in the depths of your subconscious as well as the patterns held in the 'junk DNA'.

The usual instruction is to tap each point seven times in a specific sequence of three rounds. But you will find that you quickly move into your own rhythm cycle as your intuition takes over. It may feel quite confusing when you first start tapping and saying your set-up statement at the same time, but that's OK. It's part of why it works. Tapping takes you out of your rational mind by giving that part of the brain something to focus on. This prevents the rational mind from censoring the information that arises into the intuitive mind and allows the patterns and memories in the brain to be reprinted. So, in a way, the more confused you are the better.

Tapping for the ancestors or your previous life self

One of the beauties of Crystal EFT is that you can use yourself as a surrogate and tap on your body *for the benefit of someone else* even when this is a past life persona or an ancestor. So, if you know that there is a specific person who was the source of an ancestral issue or trans-generational trauma, you can tap as though you were that person. Or you can tap on yourself as you were in a former life. But, if you do not know the source, you can also tap more generally for the ancestral line, or yourself, as a whole.

The tapping points

Crystal EFT adds chakras to the conventional EFT tapping points – and you can add others such as the base, navel, sacral or solar plexus if this feels appropriate. Never hesitate to go where your intuition and the crystal directs your hand. For karmic and ancestral work, you can tap the past life chakras that run from the back of the ears down to the hollow in the base of your skull. If two points are illustrated, tap whichever side of your face is easiest – you do not have to tap on both sides, nor do you have to follow the order rigidly. The more you can go with the flow the better. Tap with whichever hand feels most comfortable. You can switch in the middle if that feels better.

While formulating your set-up statement (see below), tap for as long as you rant. Don't try to keep count of the taps or to censor what you say, just tap the top of your head or the side of your hand and allow the words to come out. When you have your set-up statement and shorthand statements, each point is then tapped seven times or thereabouts. Do what feels right for you. There may be times when your hand wants to reverse the direction, moving back up from the spleen chakra to the past life chakras on your head, for instance, or going down to the chakras in your lower body. Carrying out at least three rounds of tapping, becoming more positive with each round, allows you to fully feel the effect; but once again 'going with the flow' attunes to how you need to do it, and you may do a particular round several times or only once.

You may need to tap again later if something deeper surfaces as you will have released an obstructing layer so that core issues or patterns can emerge. The past life chakras are particularly relevant for this. Other places on your body may also call out to be tapped, such as either side of the breastbone about a hand's breadth below the collarbone. These points are known as 'spirit ground' in Chinese medicine and assist with the pain of being in incarnation and also with releasing emotional pain. Tapping these points calls your spirit home to your physical body and helps to release the pain. All the chakras could be tapped as they hold ancestral and karmic issues that may need releasing. Go with your intuition and be guided by the crystal.

Illustration 2: The tapping points. NB: Where points are shown on each side of the face, choose one side or the other to tap. You do not have to tap all the points. Be creative and intuitive when you tap. Do what feels right for you!

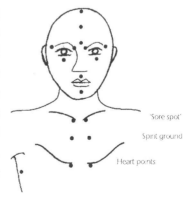

'Sore spot'

Spirit ground

Heart points

The tapping points

- **'Karate chop':** the outer edge of the hand. Tap with all fingers of other hand with the crystal in your palm.
- **Crown chakra:** top of the head. Tap with crystal.
- **Soma chakra:** centre of the forehead at the hairline. Tap with crystal.
- **Third eye:** centre of the forehead slightly above the eyebrows. Tap with crystal.
- **Inner corner of the eyebrow:** Tap with crystal.
- **Outer corner of the eyebrow:** Tap one with crystal.
- **Below the centre of the eye:** Tap with crystal.
- **Below the nose:** Tap with crystal.
- **Centre of the chin:** Tap with crystal.
- **'Sore spot':** on collarbone either side of the breastbone. Tap with thumb and fingers either side or alternate tapping each side with the crystal.
- **Spleen chakra:** under the left armpit. Tap with all fingers or crystal.

Additional point for karmic work:

- **Past life chakras:** along the bony ridge of the skull. Tap with crystal from just behind your ear along the bony ridge to the hollow at the back of your neck. Then proceed to the back of the other ear. Reverse the process and tap back towards the first ear. You can complete the process by moving up to the crown chakra if this feels appropriate.

Useful points for transgenerational work:

- **Past life chakras:** as above.
- **Base and sacral chakras and the navel:** at the base of your belly and just below your navel or around the navel. Tap with crystal over your clothes or gently on bare skin.

Useful points for emotional or spiritual pain:

- **Heart points:** tap either side of your breastbone about a hand's breadth beneath your collarbone (just above the breasts in women and slightly higher than the nipples in men). It is usual to tap these points with all the fingers on one side and the thumb on the other, but you can tap up and down each side with a crystal.
- **Solar plexus:** tap over your solar plexus with the point of the crystal – use over clothes.

The set-up statement

Crystal EFT begins with crystal tapping during a stream of consciousness rant out of which a 'set-up statement' emerges. This should be made as black and negative as possible. Say out loud everything that comes into your head and don't be afraid to exaggerate it so that it is deeply negative and totally pessimistic. Hidden, unconscious beliefs, toxic thoughts and emotions will surface and be absorbed by the crystal. There may be enormous anger, hurt, jealousy or loneliness; or a deep sense of lack that has no name. This rant identifies the core issues you are going to tap on. It will be transformed as you tap.

So you could, for instance, rant about being sabotaged just at the point where your life is about to change. A typical rant would be: *"Never actually moving forward, meeting too many obstacles. Everyone else gets the breaks. Someone always puts the boot in. The world has it in for me, always has, always will. I'll never amount to anything. I'm just not good enough. No one in the family made good. I'm just like my mum. She held me back. Wouldn't let me go to uni, said I'd get married and it would be wasted. She didn't do anything with her life. Nor her mum before her. Little women, living little lives. Never amounting to anything…"* You may quickly come to recognise that this is something to do with living out your mother's fears for you, and that this came out of her own blocked ambitions and fears for herself, which in turn went back to her mother and so on. If you know the family history, you may identify that this pattern goes way back through the matrilineal line. And, if you know your own karmic history, you may find that it is a deeply ingrained pattern in your previous lives too. So, your set-up statement in this case would be: "Even though I'm following the same old patterns from my matriarchal [and karmic] line, getting sabotaged, never getting where I want to go, failing miserably, full of fear etc, etc, *nevertheless I deeply and completely love, accept and forgive myself and my matriarchal line.*"

Your personal set-up statement is always followed by:

> *Nevertheless I deeply and completely love, accept and forgive myself* [and my matriarchal/patriarchal/ancestral line if appropriate].

No matter what your personal statement may be, no matter how black, **this is the phrase you always add at the end.** It is the key to karmic, ancestral and emotional healing. Using a crystal supports you in forgiving and loving yourself deeply and your ancestral line fully and unconditionally. Crystals are love solidified, and a crystal joyfully transfers that love to you.

Once you have established the set-up statement, find a word or two to sum it up and repeat that as you tap, allowing it to evolve and change as you do so.

The tapping process

First round

- *Chose a word or phrase that is shorthand for your issue (in the example above it could be: 'sabotaged', 'held back', 'failing' or 'fear of the future'). It will change as you move through the points, so allow whatever needs to be said to come out of your mouth. Reassure yourself that there is no one right way to do tapping and no right thing to say. You can do and say whatever works for you.*
- *Then start the three rounds of tapping the points in*

whatever sequence feels right to you whilst allowing your set-up statement to evolve and become more positive. Many people start with the side of the hand and then move to the head and down the body, but this is not mandatory. Remember that counting the taps is part of the process to keep your brain occupied and it will get easier once you find your own natural rhythm.

- *As you tap, let your thoughts and feelings flow freely, simply say whatever comes to mind without censoring or judging; it will change as it is uncovered and tapped. With each round of tapping, the statement will become more positive and life affirming, creating change and transformation in your 'junk DNA' and in the brain.*
- *Cleanse your crystal if this feels appropriate.*

Second and third rounds

- *Rephrase your initial set-up statement to allow for change and become more positive.*
- *Do several rounds of tapping if necessary until your final statement is completely positive. (In the example above it could be 'taking charge of my life, making a success of it, fulfilling my potential'.)*
- *'Karate chop' the side of your hand, the top of your head or your past life chakras seven times or so whilst repeating the new statement out loud, again allowing any changes or unconscious phrases to be spoken. End with:*

"And I deeply and completely love, accept and forgive myself" [and...]

Finally

- *Sit quietly for a few moments reviewing how you feel and enjoying the change you have brought about. If you are using a Brandenberg, place it over your heart as you do this.*

You will know that the Crystal EFT has worked when you stop attracting into your life situations, and people, who mirrored or provoked those olds fears, toxic emotions, obsessive thoughts; and your ancestral or karmic patterns no longer override your soul intention. But, until you do, keep tapping on any issues and feelings that emerge, bearing in mind that they are helping you to get to the bottom of things and transform in the depths of your being. Literally, reprogramming your 'junk DNA' (see page 91). Having said that, Crystal EFT can work amazingly fast, especially when you hold the intention of letting go and transforming.

Do not feel that it hasn't worked or that you 'got it wrong' if you do find yourself back in the old pattern; this is merely a sign that you need to uncover a deeper issue. Go back into the stream of consciousness, exaggerate the negativity that is rising, and allow whatever lies in the deepest recesses of your mind and 'junk DNA' to surface and transform. Tap on whatever comes up. Always remembering to follow with the key phrase:

> *Nevertheless I deeply and completely love, accept and forgive myself.*

[Extracted and adapted from *Good Vibrations*]

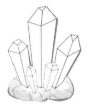

Finding Your Prescription

A choice of crystal prescriptions is offered under each entry in the A–Z Directory. This is because each person's energy field with its ancestral and karmic history is unique. As is the ancestral timeline. So, you need to match crystals with your particular field rather than using a 'one size fits all' template. Some crystals have a much finer vibration than others, working from the subtle ancestral or karmic blueprint to adjust the physical body and 'junk DNA'. Earthy, lower vibration crystals operate at the physical level first to effect permanent changes in the 'junk DNA', the cells of the physical body, and then the karmic blueprint. Other

Higher and lower vibration crystals

The description 'higher' and 'lower' vibration reflects the resonance frequency of a crystal. 'Lower' vibrations have a denser, more earthy and physical frequency than the more cosmic higher vibration crystals.

crystals operate more subtly, frequently bringing under-lying causes to the surface for resolution, so that you may need to use a series of crystals.

You may find that you are instinctively drawn to a particular stone. If so, try this one first. The best way to select your crystals for ancestral and karmic clearing, and for soul retrieval, is to choose them intuitively. Allowing your fingers to instinctively pick the right stone from a number of stones – usually the one that 'sticks' to them, gives excellent results, and or the one to which your eye is drawn. But you can also dowse for crystals (see below). You may be able to utilise what you already have in your crystal toolkit as we tend to be attracted to crystals that have something to offer us.

Framing your questions

The issues in ancestral and karmic clearing tend to be both subtle and complex so framing your question when dowsing for the most beneficial crystal requires careful thought (see page 117). Questions need to be unambiguous and capable of a straight 'yes' or 'no' answer. Take time to prepare yourself. Sit quietly for a few moments, bringing your focus away from the outside world and quietening your mind. Word your question carefully. If, for instance, you ask: "Is this the right crystal for me?" the answer could well be 'yes', but may indicate a crystal that could well be of value to you in the long term, but it may not be the most appropriate starting point at which to peel back the layers. You need to be specific: "Am I suffering from soul loss?" "Is there an ancestral pattern at work here?" "Is there an underlying karmic issue?" If so, see below on dowsing the A–Z Directory.

On the other hand, being too specific could be limiting shutting off wider possibilities. Staying flexible and exploring possibilities rather than assuming that you know the answer before you receive it is necessary. It is essential to clear your mind before asking questions.

If you are finger dowsing (see page 121), you could ask: "Is [name of crystal] the best and most appropriate crystal to heal my ancestral line at this time?" for instance. Or, "Is [name of crystal] the best one to help me free myself from abuse in the past." If you are pendulum dowsing (see page 118), ask: "Please show me the best and most appropriate crystal for [issue] now." Move your hand over the list of crystals or the crystals themselves as you do so. It could also be worthwhile enquiring: "Is there a deeper condition underlying this issue?" If the answer is 'yes', ask: "Does this condition lie at the physical [wait for a moment for the pendulum to respond], emotional [wait for a moment], mental [wait for a moment], karmic [wait for a moment], ancestral [wait for a moment] or soul [wait for a moment], or spiritual level?"

Dowsing the Directory

You can either use a pendulum when choosing crystals or finger dowse. Both methods use the ability of your intuitive body-mind connection to tune into subtle vibrations and to influence your hands. A focused mind, trust in the process, carefully worded questions and a clear intent support your dowsing and your healing.

Pendulum

If you are familiar with pendulum dowsing, use the pendulum in your usual way. If you are not, this skill is easily learned.

To pendulum dowse

To pendulum dowse, hold your pendulum between the thumb and forefinger of your most receptive hand with about a hand's length of chain hanging down to the pendulum – you will soon learn what is the right length for you. Wrap the remaining chain around your fingers so that it does not obstruct the dowsing.

You will need to ascertain which is a 'yes' and which is a 'no' response. Some people find that the pendulum swings in one direction for 'yes' and at right angles to that axis for 'no', while others have a backwards and forwards swing for one reply, and a circular motion for the other. A 'wobble' of the pendulum can indicate a 'maybe' or that it is not appropriate to dowse at that time, or that the wrong question is being asked. In which case, ask if it is appropriate, and if the answer is 'yes', check that you are framing the question in the correct way. If the pendulum stops completely it is usually inappropriate to ask at that time.

You can ascertain your particular pendulum response by holding the pendulum over your knee and asking: "Is my name [correct name]?" The direction that the pendulum swings will indicate 'yes'. Check by asking: "Is my name [incorrect name]?" to establish 'no'. Or, you can programme in 'yes' and 'no' by swinging the pendulum in a particular direction a few times, saying as you do: "This is yes", and swinging it in a different direction to programme in 'no'.

To pendulum dowse the best crystal for you

To ascertain which crystal will be most beneficial for you, hold the pendulum in your most receptive hand. Put the forefinger of your other hand on the condition or issue. Slowly run your finger along the list of possible crystals, noting whether you get a 'yes' or 'no' response. Check the whole list to see which 'yes' response is strongest as there may well be several that would be appropriate or you may need to use several crystals in combination. Another way to do this, if you have several of the crystals available, is to touch each crystal in turn, again noting the 'yes' or 'no' response.

If you get a no response when checking out the issue, touch each of the capital letters in turn until you receive a yes, then run your finger down the entries in that section.

How long should I use a crystal?

A pendulum can also be used to establish how long a

crystal should be left in place. This is particularly useful if you are placing the crystal over or around your body or bed, but it can also be helpful if you are wearing a crystal and need to know whether or not to wear it at night – in which case you will get a 'yes' or 'no' answer to the question: "Should I remove this crystal at night?" To establish timing, use an arc on which you have marked five-minute or one-hour or one-day intervals (ask in advance whether the period should be checked in minutes, hours or days). Hold the hand with the pendulum over the centre of the arc and ask that the pendulum will go towards the correct period (see illustration).

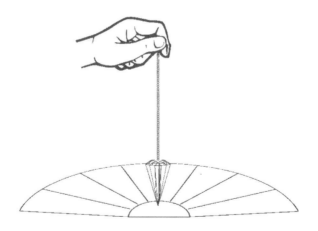

Dowsing over an Arc

Finger Dowsing

Finger dowsing answers 'yes' and 'no' questions quickly and unambiguously, and can be done unobtrusively in situations where a pendulum might provoke unwanted attention. This method of dowsing works particularly well for people who are kinaesthetic, that is to say their body responds intuitively to subtle feelings, but anyone can learn to finger dowse.

To finger dowse

To finger dowse, hold the thumb and first finger of your right hand together (see illustration). Loop the thumb and finger of your left hand through to make a 'chain'. Ask your question clearly and unambiguously – you can speak it aloud or keep it within your mind. Now pull gently but firmly. If the chain breaks, the answer is 'no'. If it holds, the answer is 'yes'.

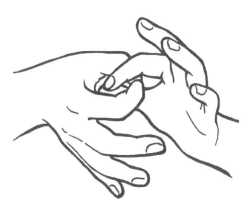

To finger dowse timing

Questions such as "Should I leave the crystal in place overnight" can be answered by the usual finger dowsing method, although you should follow up a 'yes' answer with the question "And longer?" to ascertain whether further time may be appropriate. Asking about periods of time requires a slightly different method. First, ask whether the period required is minutes, hours, days, weeks or months. When you have ascertained the answer, slot your fingers together and ask that they will hold until the right answer is reached and then release. You can then ask, "1 minute, 2 minutes," and so on, or 1 hour/day/month until you have a definitive answer.

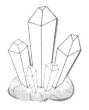

Crystal Care

Purifying Your Crystal

Crystals need regular cleansing, purifying and recharging. This is particularly so when they are being used for healing or clearing. It is sensible to purify and re-energize a crystal every time it is used. The method employed will depend on the type of crystal. Soft and friable crystals, for instance, and those that are attached to a base can be damaged by water, and soft stones such as Halite will dissolve. These are best purified by a 'dry' process such as brown rice and recharged sunlight, but sturdier crystals benefit from being placed under running water or in the sea. Crystals work best when their energy is harnessed and focused with intent towards the task at hand as this activates them. By taking the time to attune a crystal to your own unique frequency, you enhance its vibratory effect and amplify its healing power. But do not limit it, ask "… this or something better."

Methods:

Running water

Hold your crystals under a running tap, or, preferably, pour spring water over them, or place them in a stream or the ocean to draw off negative energy (use a bag to hold small crystals). You can also immerse appropriate crystals in a bowl of water into which a handful of sea salt or rock salt has been added. (Salt is best avoided if the crystal is layered or friable.) Dry the crystal carefully afterwards and place in the sun to re-energize.

Rice or salt

Place your crystal in a bowl of salt or brown rice and leave overnight for the negative energies to be absorbed. (Brush salt off carefully and make sure that it has been removed from any niches or cracks in the crystal as otherwise it will absorb water in the future and could cause splintering.) Place the crystals in the sun to re-energize.

Smudging

Sage, sweetgrass or joss sticks are excellent for smudging as they quickly remove negative energies. Light the smudge stick and pass it over the crystal if it is large, or hold the crystal in your hand in the smoke if it is small. It is traditional to fan the smoke gently with a feather but this is not essential.

Visualising light

Hold your crystal in your hands and visualise a column of bright white light coming down and covering the crystal, absorbing anything negative it may have picked up and restoring the pure energy once more. If you find visualisation difficult, you can use the light of a candle.

Sound

Tuning forks, singing bowls or tingshaws can also be used to cleanse a crystal but the crystal will then require recharging.

Crystal clearing essences

A number of crystal clearing and recharging essences are available from flower essence suppliers, crystal shops and the Internet (see Resources). You can either drop the essence directly on to the crystal, gently rubbing it over the crystal with your finger, or put a few drops into clean spring water in an atomiser or spray bottle and gently mist the crystal.

Re-Energizing Your Crystal

Crystals can be placed on a Quartz cluster or on a large Carnelian to re-energize them but the light of the sun is an excellent energizer. Red and yellow crystals particularly enjoy being placed in the sun, and white and pale-coloured crystals respond well to the moon. (Be aware that sunlight focused through a crystal may be a fire hazard, and delicate crystals will lose their colour quickly if left exposed to light.) Some brown crystals, such as Smoky Quartz, respond to being placed on or in the earth. If you bury a crystal, remember to mark its position clearly.

Focusing and Activating Your Crystal

Once your crystal has been purified and re-energized, sit quietly holding the crystal in your hands for a few minutes until you feel in tune with it. Picture it surrounded by light and love. State that the crystal is dedicated to the highest good of all who use it. Then state very clearly your intention for the crystal – that it will heal or protect you, for instance. If it is intended for a specific purpose such as healing a particular condition, state that also. But remember to add "this or something better". Repeat the intention several times to anchor it into the crystal.

Deprogramming a Crystal

There may be times when a crystal has been dedicated for one particular use but is no longer required for that purpose. This does not mean its usefulness is over. It will undoubtedly have other work to do and another purpose to carry out. It is therefore sensible to deprogramme a crystal and put a new intention in before using it again.

To deprogramme a crystal

Hold the crystal in your hands for a few moments, thanking it for doing its work and for holding the intention and purpose it has had. Explain to the crystal that this part of its work is now over and ask the crystal to dismantle the programme it has been carrying. See bright white light beaming into the crystal to help it to deprogramme, cleanse and recharge. Wash the crystal in Clear2Light and/or Z14 or other cleansing spray, or place it under running water. Put the crystal out into sunlight for a few hours or under the moon. The crystal may need a rest period to rebuild its energies before being rededicated to a new purpose.

If you are not visual: Cleanse the crystal with Clear2Light, place it under running water or into brown rice, or use tingshaws or a Tibetan bowl, and then leave in sunlight or moonlight for a few hours. Then place the crystal on a Brandenberg Quartz and ask that it be returned to its original pure vibrations. Leave overnight. Then remove the crystal and allow it to rest before being rededicated.

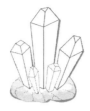

Using Your Crystals for Healing

Are not gross Bodies and Light convertible into one another, and may not Bodies receive much of their Activity from the Particles of Light which enter their Composition? The changing of Bodies into Light, and Light into Bodies, is very conformable to the Course of Nature, which seems delighted with Transmutations.
Sir Isaac Newton, *Principia*

Most crystals can be placed over clothing on a chakra or energy meridian, or the site of dis-ease, and left in place for 15–20 minutes or so. They can also be placed around the body, out in the aura or in your space to create energetic grids. Crystals work well placed in the aura about a foot out from the physical body as that is where many of the more subtle imprints, engrams, attachments and influences occur. Sweeping the whole aura with an appropriate crystal such as Anandalite often clears minor issues without the need to have further insight or information. If you are working with the ancestors, crystals can be placed on photographs or on the family tree.

If your crystal has a point, place it point towards

yourself, or point down if placed on your body, to draw healing or re-energizing properties into your body. Place it point out, or point down below your feet to draw off imprints, attachments, toxic residues or emotional debris. When you have placed the stones, close your eyes and breathe gently and evenly, and allow yourself to relax and feel the energy of the crystal radiating out through your whole being. If you are working on the ancestors or past lives, picture the crystal energy flowing way back into the past and then coming forward to bring healing up to the present moment and beyond into future generations.

You can also apply crystal essences (see pages 131–135). These essences convey crystal vibes to the body at a subtle level and are particularly effective for emotional conditions and for assimilating high vibrational downloads and making soul shifts or reintegrations.

Healing challenge

Occasionally crystals trigger a 'healing challenge' when symptoms appear to get worse rather than better and flu-like symptoms may occur, or a member of the family will act-out, intensely repeating the old pattern. This is an indication of physical, emotional, mental, karmic or ancestral toxins leaving the body and is all part of the body holistically healing itself. It occurs particularly in stress-related or chronic conditions. It can be soothed and facilitated by crystals such as Smoky Elestial Quartz,

Eye of the Storm or Quantum Quattro, and by drinking plenty of water (Shungite-infused water is ideal). If a healing challenge occurs, use these stones for a few days until the symptoms dissipate and then return to the crystals you were using – having dowsed or intuited if they are still appropriate.

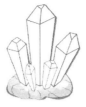

Crystal Essences

Crystal essences are an excellent way to use the healing power of crystals, and several crystals can be combined provided you dowse to check compatibility. The essence can be gently rubbed on the skin over a chakra, or dripped on to a crystal placed on an ancestral photograph. Essences can also be added to a glass of water and sipped, or taken from a dropper bottle, or spritzed around the aura (add seven drops to spring water in a spray bottle). Crystal essences are made by transferring the subtle energies and minute concentrations of the mineral constituents of the crystal into water except where a crystal may be toxic; see Contraindications in the Directory – in which case use the indirect method. The water stores the vibrations and transfers them to the chakras, physical or subtle bodies in exactly the same way that a homoeopathic essence works. The essence is bottled and a preservative – brandy, vodka or cider vinegar – added. If the essence is to be taken by those for whom alcohol is inappropriate, cider vinegar can be used as a preservative or the essence rubbed on the skin. (See Resources for purpose-made highly effective essences.)

Caution: Some stones contain trace minerals that are toxic (see the list in Contraindications) and essences from these stones need to be made by an indirect method that transfers the vibrations without transferring any of the toxic material from the stone (see page 133). If in doubt, make the essence by the indirect method, which is also suitable for fragile or layered stones. Always wash your hands after handling these stones and use in a tumbled version wherever possible.

Making a Crystal Essence

You will need the appropriate crystal, which has been cleansed and purified (see pages 123–125), one or two clean glass bowls, spring water and a suitable bottle in which to keep the essence (coloured glass is preferable to clear as it preserves the vibrations better). Essences can be made by the direct or indirect method. The indirect method is suitable for friable, layered or clustered crystals as well as those that may have a degree of toxicity. Spring water should be used rather than tap water that has chlorine, fluoride and aluminium added to it. Water from a spring with healing properties is particularly effective.

Direct method

Place enough spring water in a glass bowl to just cover the crystal. Stand the bowl in sunlight for several hours.

(If the bowl is left outside, cover with a glass lid or cling film to prevent insects falling into it.) If appropriate, the bowl can also be left overnight in moonlight.

Indirect method

If the crystal is toxic or fragile (see Contraindications page 301) place the crystal in a small glass bowl and stand the bowl within a large bowl that has sufficient spring water to raise the level above the crystal in the inner bowl. Stand the bowl in sunlight for several hours. (If the bowl is left outside, cover with a glass lid or cling film.) If appropriate, the bowl can also be left overnight in moonlight.

Bottling and preserving

If the essence is not to be used within a day or two, top up with two-thirds brandy, vodka, white rum or cider vinegar to one-third essence, otherwise the essence may become musty. This makes a 'mother tincture' that can be further diluted. To make a small dosage bottle, add seven drops of the mother essence to a dosage bottle containing two-thirds brandy and one-third water. If a spray bottle is being made, add seven drops of mother essence to pure water if using immediately. For prolonged use, vodka or white rum make a useful preservative as they have no smell.

Using a crystal essence

For short-term use, an essence can be sipped every few

minutes, rubbed on the appropriate chakra, or placed on a crystal. Hold the water in your mouth for a few moments if taking orally. For longer term use, take three times a day. Essences can also be applied to the skin, either at the wrist or over the site of a problem, or added to bath water. If a spray bottle is made, add seven drops of the essence to spring water and spritz around the aura (front and back), over a grid or appropriate chakras, remembering that these may extend for several feet out from the physical body.

Shungite water

Shungite water is an extremely effective healer, both at a physical and subtle level. To become biologically active, water needs to have Shungite immersed in it for at least 48 hours. However, once the first batch has been made, you may simply refill the filter jug every time you use some of the water so that it is constantly replenished. Wash the jug and the bag of Shungite at least once a week depending on how much water you have used (you can store the activated water and return it to the jug). Place the Shungite in the sun or fresh air for a few hours to recharge, or use a proprietary crystal cleansing and recharging essence. Raw Shungite is more effective than the tumbles, but, no matter how often the non-vitreous type of Shungite has been washed and the use of a fine mesh bag, it will leave a very fine suspension of black particles in the water. This is all part of the healing process.

Making the water:

You will need:
2-litre filter jug
Fine mesh 2″ bag of raw Shungite (10–100gm)

Place the mesh bag of Shungite in the base of the filter jug (if using tap water you can also use a commercial filter if the jug is provided with one). Pour water into the jug until it is full. Stand it aside for 48 hours. Then top up the water each time it is used.

Cleanse the Shungite frequently under running water and re-energize in the sun or fresh air.

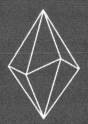

Part II
Karmic Healing

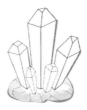

A blast from the past

Past life regression allows people to travel back in time, to release energy patterns no longer serving them, and to discover sources of knowledge they once knew and draw upon the wellspring of information stored deep within the soul... stones will help you by bridging the gap between the blueprint of perfection in your holographic self with the physical shell you find yourself in today.

Past Lives with Gems & Stones, Shelley Kaehr

Old karma. There's a lot of it hanging about. Some of it is yours – and some of it is mine. But some of it belongs to neither of us. Huge chunks attach to the ancestors and pass down the ancestral line. It's what we call collective and transgenerational. Other karma can be attached to land, to a racial group or to humanity itself. To war, conflict and enslavement. To abuse and misuse of power – and of the environment. It is part of a collective karmic enmeshment. But it's become the forgotten karma. No one person is responsible for creating it. Nevertheless, we all have a share in it. It's part of history. Yet it needs to be cleansed. If we are going to shift into a new vibrational frequency, then we have to release from the karmic past, personal or otherwise. There's no way we can drag it with us into the expanded consciousness of the Age of Aquarius. Shame and guilt, victimhood and martyrdom, judgementalism and sacrifice, bigoted minds and outdated beliefs belong to the Age of Pisces and that's passing into history. This is a pivotal, axial moment. It's time for a revitalisation – and an Aquarian realisation that another option is opening up, that of healing and forgiveness.

> *Beliefs are a form of self-hypnosis. They are the guiding fictions which we repeat to ourselves so often, and with such conviction, that we forget that they are simply themes in a script we have written, and act as if they were true. "Life is full of suffering", we might tell ourselves – and we see confirmation of our belief in every conversation with our problem-ridden friends, with every disaster-obsessed news report (which we compulsively listen to), and with every fresh trauma and misfortune that we attract into our own lives.*
> Gill Edwards

Our karma is literally a blast from the past. Something beyond our conscious control that kicks in and overwhelms us. A series of beliefs, imprints, patterns and suppositions created from past experience or inherited from the ancestral line. It is carried in the karmic blueprint, the 'junk DNA', the psoas muscle and our minds. Soul imperatives, or overlays, together with engrams (see page 145) are deeply ingrained patterns, reactions or intentions laid down over many lifetimes which may well have been outgrown but not shed by the soul, and which compel certain behaviour no matter how much the soul may wish to override them. Unless cleared, they distort the soul's intention, pulling it back into outdated ways of being. Such scripts are made up of all the 'oughts, shoulds and musts', conditioned responses and expectations arising from the past, whenever that might be. Changing a soul imperative can bring about a profound level of healing. One of the simplest ways of working with a crystal to heal the past is to identify, and then release, the soulscripts or karmic imprints that you carry either by taking an appropriate crystal essence or by using the crystals themselves in grids, placements and layouts.

Typical soulscripts and engrams

Unworthiness	Undeservedness	Guilt
Aggression	Fear	Sadness
Self-doubt	Self-sabotage	Wounded self
Shame	Martyrdom	'Poor me'
Perfectionism	People-pleasing	Terrorist
Poverty Consciousness	Addiction	Sorcerer
Emotional vampire	Care-giver	Tyrant
Victim-Persecutor-Rescuer	Failure	Hedonist
Codependency	Sybarite	Control freak
Disempowered	Addict	Dispossessed

Judgemental	Self-righteous	God-complex
Madonna	Whore	Servant
Entitlement	Master	Saviour
Defensive	Overly-detached	Profligate
Rebellious	Fantasist	Puer
Suffering	Hero	Hysteric
Drama Queen	Miser	Obsession

Karmic clearing

Soulscripts can quickly be dissolved by placing appropriate crystals on and around the body, especially on the chakras. You can use your own body as a surrogate for an ancestor if necessary or use a photograph if you have one. By choosing a crystal that resonates with a known script or issue, you can restore balance to the subtle bodies and imprint a new, more positive pattern. The effect then filters into the physical. However, when a script has not yet been recognised, placing past life crystals allows it to float to the surface and be transmuted without necessarily knowing all the details. (See also Healing 'junk DNA' in Part I.)

The figure of eight layout is especially helpful, bringing, as it does, the causal vortex with its connection to the Akashic Record closer to conscious awareness and grounding the resulting change into the physical body. The core layout can be expanded by adding appropriate crystals over the chakras. When the stones have been laid, join up the figure of eight with a crystal wand or the power of your mind.

General Clearing grid

- *Lie down and place a grounding stone at your feet opposite the causal vortex point.*
- *Place Anandalite or a causal vortex crystal on the causal vortex (see page 53).*
- *Place a unification and integration crystal over the dantien.*
- *Join up the grid with a crystal wand or the power of your mind.*
- *Place appropriate crystals on the chakras as required.*

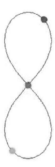

The core layout: Anandalite on the causal vortex, Flint or Smoky Quartz at the feet, and a unification stone over the dantien.

To clear the mind and third eye of past life imprints and embargos

- *Lie down comfortably and open your grounding root (see page 19).*
- *Open the causal vortex with an appropriate crystal (see page 292).*

- *Place an Auralite 23 point down above your head.*
- *Place Bytownite, Rhomboid Selenite or other third eye crystal on your third eye.*
- *Place a Preseli Bluestone on your soma chakra.*
- *Place a past life chakra stone on either side of your head level with your ears.*
- *If it feels appropriate, place a past life clearing stone or piece of Flint under the hollow at the base of your skull.*
- *Allow the crystals to cleanse the chakras and remove any imprints and memories from your mind and third eye. Do not seek to see any past lives, simply be willing to let go.*
- *When the session is complete, remove and thoroughly cleanse the crystals and close the chakras by imaging shutters folding over them or placing an appropriate crystal.*
- *Check that your grounding cord is in place.*

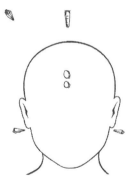

Mind clearing past life healing layout

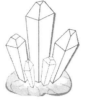

Death and the Afterlife

Now if it be true that the living come from the dead, then our souls must exist in the other world, for if not how could they have been born again?
Socrates

Before we go any further with karmic clearing it may be helpful to look at the soul's journey after death and before incarnation. Karmic healing presupposes that a soul – or family of souls – has lived before in a physical or other subtle form and has returned, from the multidimensional realms, into earthly incarnation carrying with it the subtle imprints, memory traces or engrams and the karmas of previous experience. The soul can reincarnate again at any of the stages below once the 'silver cord' that holds the etheric bodies to the physical has been severed. If the soul is pulled quickly back into incarnation, it will take on its old emotions and unlived-out desires, engrams and imprints. Such an incarnation may not be purposeful, other than to follow the old pattern or fulfil addictions and obsessions. If the soul moves beyond the mental planes and into the spiritual planes, and goes through a healing and insight process, then the next incarnation is more likely to be well planned and purposeful, although old vows and promises may pull it back to be with another soul again, or to work on unfinished business.

Engram
An engram is a mental image or memory trace that records an experience containing pain, trauma, locked emotions and attitudes, unconsciousness and a real or fancied threat to survival. An engram can be created in a past life and carried over to the present through the karmic blueprint and subtle DNA.

The Stages of Death and Reincarnation

1   The soul/consciousness detaches from the physical as the 'silver cord' severs.
2   Subtle bodies and the soul leave the physical, taking embedded engrams and imprints.
3   Life Review – the soul re-experiences old emotions, recognises lessons and gains insights.
4   Move into an astral body. The soul may live out unexperienced desires on the etheric plane. This is where many people bounce back into incarnation, pulled back by unfinished business or overwhelming desires, bringing engrams and imprints back into incarnation. Or, the soul may

go on to heal past traumas.

5   Moving on, the soul detaches from desires and moves into the mental body to review ideas, beliefs and constructs, and seek understanding of the gifts in an experience. If not reframed, subtle engrams and imprints may be carried over.

6   Moving to a higher level, the soul detaches from old beliefs and ideals. It receives 'higher mind' teachings and expands awareness.

7   The soul moves into the spiritual body to undergo necessary healing and obtain further insights. Decisions are formulated that are not simply a repetition of karmic patterns.

8   Decision to return is made in the between (inter) life state.

9   The soul attends a planning meeting and formulates a life plan – if this stage is skipped, old patterns and interactions will simply be repeated. Parents, partners, children and life circumstances are chosen. Reconnection is made to old skills and emotions.

10   The soul moves into the etheric body. A new physical body is created from the etheric and karmic blueprint and the imprints and engrams therein.

11   Conception occurs. Ancestral imprints and engrams are added through DNA.

12   Intrauterine experience and birth process reactivates old emotional, karmic, ancestral and mental patterns.

13   Birth into new incarnation.

[For more information see *The Book of Why*.]

Between (inter) life state

The 'holding space' that a soul inhabits between physical incarnations. Often initially experienced according to cultural or religious beliefs, the interlife has many planes of experience. Time as we know it on Earth does not operate. The soul occupies a less dense 'body' – although it may have a similar appearance. To the soul, this space is solid and tangible. Healing and reframing can easily be carried out in the interlife and a soul's purpose ascertained. Souls spend an indefinite period in the between life state until ready to return to Earth when a 'planning meeting' usually takes place to prepare for the new life.

Reframing

Reframing changes the lifescript or engram for a particular incarnation. It may entail a change of scenario, replaying it with a different outcome. It may need to be seen from a different perspective or with forgiveness or compassionate witnessing. Changing the past in this way changes the present life experience.

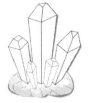

Choosing a new incarnation

In the days before I knew of pre-birth planning, I felt sympathy for others who appeared to be less fortunate than I, pitying a homeless person on the street, for example. Now aware that this seemingly 'bad' experience may have been planned, I feel only deep respect.

Robert Schwartz, *Courageous Souls*

New incarnations are planned whilst in the between life state at what I call "the planning meeting". At this meeting a lifeplan is prepared. Contacts, contracts and events are sketched out and a rough timing schedule mapped (see *The Book of Why*). From past life work with people over many years, it would appear that most souls have at least a modicum of choice, although some people do not progress far enough in the between life state to make an informed choice. They either simply 'bounce back' into incarnation because of strong desires – for a substance, experience or person; or they are pulled back by ingrained patterns or old promises or vows that have not been rescinded. The major challenge for the present life may be to break the habits of lifetimes, or to release someone – or oneself – from an outdated promise or an ancestral engram passed down the family line. People who incarnate without planning or preparation go around and around on the wheel of karma.

On the other hand, someone who may appear to be 'fated', because of trauma or dis-ease, may have made that choice deliberately. Choices that are, at first glance, surprising may have been made for soul growth to learn specific qualities. Illness or traumatic life situations may have been prepared most carefully for the incarnation, and the soul may have a profound reason for making that choice. It may be for personal growth and learning, or to facilitate other people in their lessons or intentions.

The Lifeplan

The lifeplan is not rigid. It is an outline rather than a line by line account of how the life will go. It is adaptable but has structure. The soul chooses a family situation that will reiterate attitudes, experiences or lessons from the past which the soul wants to confront or heal. The life plan will have 'key moments' mapped in so that karmic meetings or fateful decisions occur. It may also incorporate a point when previous life memories will become conscious once more to aid the soul in its evolution.

Or both. For example, someone speaking on the radio the other day said that her autistic son was teaching her patience and tolerance. Before she'd had him, she had, in her own words, been an extremely impatient, intolerant person. But, because her son appeared, to the outside world, to 'act normally' most of the time, and had no outward sign of disability, not only did she have to be patient herself with him, but had also had to negotiate with the people around him when his autism unexpectedly kicked in.

True or not true?

People ask, "Are past lives true?" But this is not the right question. Whether or not a life is actually, factually true, it will be symbolic of your soul story. Knowing the detail of your past lives can be useful as it pinpoints patterns, root causes, unfinished business, blockages, soul purpose and so on. What a past life seeing, accessing far memory or reading the Akashic Record does is to give you an overview, a picture of your soul history and that of the ancestors. What you need to ask is, "Is this true for me? Does this give me insight into myself and my family line?" However, at the end of the day, crystals can bypass the need to know and help you to simply heal.

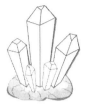

Soul groups

Simply defined – a member of your soul group is someone that has a profound, deep and intense impact on your life, whether positive or negative. The person can be in your life for five minutes or your entire life. Time is not a consideration because the things you agree to accomplish before you were born into these lives will play out as they are intended.

http://reincarnationstudies.com/resources/complexities-soul-groups/

Soul groups are groups of souls who travel together throughout timeframes and multidimensions. They set out from a 'pool' of spiritual essence that separated and combined over an infinity of time. They are loosely attached to each other and may not meet in every incarnation. When they do, it may be for surprising reasons. The person who most abuses and misuses you, for instance, may be a member of your soul group who loves you enough to support your karmic learning whatever that may be. Soul groups may include your family and ancestors, but this is by no means certain.

Soul groups are complex, intersecting and parting time and again as with the spiders' webs illustration on page 185, so that a soul may in effect belong to a soul community that consists of several soul families linked by previous interaction and group karma. A 'resonance frequency' is established between souls who have taken part in a particular soul drama so that the participants will be pulled back into incarnation at approximately the same time to heal, rework or reframe the outstanding karma from that life, in effect creating a soul group subset.

Soul group

A group of souls who have travelled together throughout time, over many incarnations, and interacted in all possible combinations. Not all members of a soul group are in incarnation at one time, but those people who help us to learn the hardest lessons in life are usually members of our primary soul group. Soul groups can split into 'subsets' that may recombine at a later date.

The emergence of a soul group. Soul A may feel disconnected from the original soul group, as may Soul D which will return to the overall 'pool' after one incarnation. They will almost certainly not recognise each other if they meet. But B and C may well recognise each other as

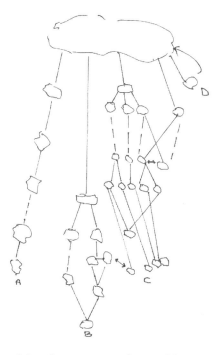

part of a soul family or as a soulmate. However, all could
potentially recognise each other as a soulmate because of
the underlying connection. Soul A has incarnated again
with a piece of soul left three lives back in the chain and
will need to reintegrate that in the present life. Soul B has
arisen from a more complex soul split. Care would need
to be taken that only appropriate parts of that soul are
called back and integrated.

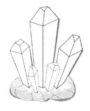

Reasons for incarnating together again

The shackles of an old love straiten'd him,
His Honour rooted in dishonour stood,
And faith unfaithful kept him falsely true.
Alfred, Lord Tennyson

As we've seen, people tend to incarnate together time and again in loosely connected soul groups. The underlying reasons can be the same whether the relationship is within the family, a group of friends, or an intimate relationship. Karma, along with soul intention, is playing itself out. I've explored this in depth in *The Soulmate Myth* and *The Book of Why*, but the reasons are briefly included here so that you can recognise them if you meet them in your ancestral or personal karmic exploration. For further understanding, however, see those books.

Positive reasons

- Spiritual bonds
- A between life decision that has to manifest

- To be soul companions or twinflames
- To facilitate soul lessons
- Lessons to be learned
- Attitudes to be transformed
- Appropriate soul contracts
- Specific tasks
- Catalyst
- Positive service

Challenging reasons

- Inappropriate soul contracts
- Previous relationship(s) carried over
- Unfinished business
- Habit or inertia
- Dependence and symbiosis
- Debt or duty
- Attachment to mutual unhappiness or happiness
- Pacts or promises
- Love or hatred
- The desire for revenge
- Enmeshment
- Guilt
- Holding on to the heart
- Illusions
- Karmic bonds
- Compulsive emotions

Indications that you have met a member of your soul group

I cannot improve on this list compiled by www.reincarnationstudies.com as it resonates totally with what I have observed from almost fifty years of attending between life planning meetings and reading birthcharts from a karmic perspective. However, I have added a final observation to the list.

Beneficial soul group traits

- They mirror or have a similar life experience as you, helping you to understand your situation better.
- They highlight your personality traits helping you to change or grow.
- They help you to turn your weaknesses into strengths.
- They help to balance out your energy and show you a different side of life.
- They help you to find patience, understanding and compassion.
- They highlight a need for you to heal or let go of certain events or emotions.
- You work together to create, brainstorm ideas or bring visions into the light.
- They come into your life to help you on your path right when you need it.
- They help to advance your soul and your soul journey.
- You work together to support global causes or a bigger vision.

- They love you enough to assist you in learning the hardest lessons, giving you a tough time when appropriate.

And I would add the challenges that can play out when the karmic treadmill is simply going around and around and people are pulled back to interact without purpose or planning, *or where two or more souls have agreed to take it to the extreme so that a breakthrough can be made.*

Challenging soul group traits

- It feels like the same old, same old – again and again.
- Attitudes and experiences are invoked that feel totally against your soul's own ethical code and belief system.
- The relationship is highly destructive.
- Intense hatred is experienced on sight.
- One person holds total power over another.
- The relationship is compulsive, obsessive, addictive and feels like 'I can't live without this person' but it brings no joy.
- One person shuns or is repelled by another.
- Members of a soul group meet again as 'soulmates' for the purpose of soul growth but the meeting may not be the joyous, trouble free union that people tend to expect from a soulmate relationship: see *The Soulmate Myth: A Dream Come True or Your Worst Nightmare?*

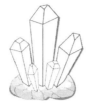

Karmic bonds and soul contracts

> *I have discovered that many troubled couples were not lovers in their former lives but enemies. In extreme cases, one partner may have even murdered the other. The person who was killed is motivated by revenge, and by marrying their killer they are in a position to do the most damage.*
> Dr Motoyama

Soul contracts are an agreement willingly – or unwittingly – made in a previous life, or in the interlife before the present incarnation, that one soul will interact with another in a specific way. Or, they may be an outdated agreement that is carried over from a previous life, or a previous interlife plan, but which has not been reconsidered before incarnation. Soul contracts can be positive and constructive, or destructive. Soul contracts that are not completed in one life may be carried over to another. Such contracts create karmic bonds and one soul may attempt to force the other to carry out a contract even when it has passed its sell-by date. Vows and promises to 'always love you/be there for you' and so on have a powerful effect beyond death, pulling the souls together again and again.

Karmic Enmeshment

Enmeshment occurs when two souls are strongly inter-twined due to previous karmic experiences. The souls incarnate together again and again in an effort to clear the situation. Enmeshment occurs when:

- relationship karma is unfulfilled or unresolved;
- the obligations to a soul for whom one is respon-sible (as in parent and child) are not fulfilled or are opted out of;
- too much responsibility is taken for someone else;
- someone who seeks their freedom is held on to;
- someone else is blamed for the soul's own limita-tions or inability to move forward;
- outdated vows, promises and soul contracts remain in force.

So often karmic enmeshment is predicated on blame, or revenge. To hold someone else culpable for the limita-tions a soul puts on itself, or a desire to be avenged, creates a situation where the souls are drawn back time and again as one struggles to become free from the other. One soul may have to learn to stop blaming the other and take responsibility. Another soul may need to forgive and let go. Another scenario that creates karmic enmeshment is where one person feeds off the other: in other words, psychic vampirism which can be energetic, emotional and monetary particularly where the vampire demands support at every level. Symbiotic, dependent relationships and situations such as master/slave or marriage where one person owns the other body and soul also create the same problem. The lesson is to let go, *even when it is passing for love.*

Enmeshment can also occur when a soul takes on too much responsibility for another – especially for their well-being or their feelings. But equally, if one soul has failed to take *appropriate* responsibility for another – as in a situation where a child is abandoned, for instance – then releasing the enmeshment may first involve appropriate parenting or care (possibly to the extent of caring for someone for an entire life if they are ill or disabled). At the right time, the soul must then be allowed the freedom to make its own journey.

Karmic enmeshment can be cleared with tie-cutting crystals, especially when these are used in conjunction with the spleen chakra release (see page 38) and a photograph of the other person is cut around with an appropriate crystal. Or, you can use the timelines exercise on page 184.

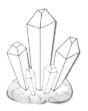

Karma

Please bear in mind that karma may apply at the ancestral level in addition to the personal. It can be transferred through soul imprints, the karmic blueprint and transgenerational 'junk DNA'. Karma is not merely what happened in the past, nor is it a fixed punishment and reward system. We create our karma and our future in every moment. Karma and time are fluid and interact with soul intention. What is created now impacts on the future and what happens in the future feeds back to affect the present. Many reported future life progressions have shown dire disaster scenarios, but also that it does not have to be that way. Progressions and regressions show that there are choices to be made at 'impact points' where timelines divide or separate, the future branches out, and different scenarios evolve. All possibilities exist *in potential* and run in the background. Indeed, at some level we may be playing them all out at once on different timelines. But your awareness will only be focused on one or two. Switch focus and you change the future you create.

Three things strongly affect karma: desire, purpose and grace:

- **Desire:** what is wanted, needed or craved creates a situation that will provide it – but this is not usually a beneficial experience. Part of the soul's lesson may be to let go of that desire and the pattern it constantly recreates. The strength of desire can transcend death and pull a soul back into incarnation to deal with unfinished business or to recreate once again a situation where the desired object can potentially be achieved. Desire creates fixed lifescripts, plans that are involuntarily followed.
- **Purpose:** what the soul needs in order to evolve. Purpose can overcome destructive desires, as when an addict goes into recovery.
- **Grace:** strengthens purpose and helps it to manifest. Grace is an offer to release karma. Grace operates when enough has been done. There are some lessons or situations that simply cannot be continued with, perhaps because of another person who is unwilling to learn or move on. Grace says that, when the soul has done all it can, it can let it go and no further karma will accrue.

So, the opportunity to create the experiences that will be most beneficial for soul growth exists. But, first, karmic dross carried from lifetime to lifetime must be released.

Karmic dross includes:

- Past-their-sell-by-date beliefs and soul imperatives
- Old vows and soul contracts
- Outdated soul purposes or lifeplans
- Entangled relationships
- Toxic emotions
- Unresolved ancestral issues
- Imprinted environmental or racial memory
- The karmic treadmill – the 'hamster wheel' effect
- Addictive patterns and habitual responses

And so much more that I have explored in *The Book of Why: Understanding Your Soul's Journey.* The remainder of this karma section is extracted from that book.

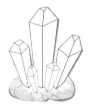

Layers and levels of karma

Karma occurs at various levels, which can override each other. Personal karma can, for instance, be dominated by transgenerational issues and ancestral themes. It may also be superseded by the needs or deeds of the collective. However, the karma of grace can override personal and collective karma. Karma does not have to be a continual round. When all that can be done has been done, or when karmic or ancestral healing takes place, the karma of grace kicks in. The souls can move on. Cosmic karma trumps all the other karmas so the need to evolve will always be the ultimate catalyst.

Karmic levels

Personal karma is carried from life to life by an individual soul. It has been created somewhere in 'the past' and the soul incarnates to deal with it in the present or to fulfil its purpose.

Ancestral karma: the karma which travels down the family line.

Group or racial karma: The group can vary in size

from a family, or group of friends or enemies, to a tribe or race or soul group. Group karma overrides individual. So, a soul who has no personal aggressive karma may nevertheless become caught up in a war or other mass movement, for instance. This is particularly so when the family carry an aggressive 'war gene' which passes into the 'junk DNA'.

Collective karma arises from all that has gone before. It is the karma of the human race. Although positive collective karma is generated, negative collective karma is what creates problems for future generations. No one is responsible for collective karma in the sense of having personally created it although individuals may, in other lives, have been part of its source in wars, purges, ideologies and other mass movements. Certain people incarnate with the intention of taking on a portion of this collective karma and clearing it for the wider whole.

Cosmic karma is the need for the whole to grow and to evolve. Cosmic karma is the spiritual purpose that can override all other karmas. It is connected to the need for each soul to evolve and to recognise, and take responsibility for, their part in the whole.

Types of karma

Merit Karma: a reward for things the soul got right in other lives, the lessons learned, the insights put into practice. It is money in the karmic piggy bank and rarely if ever needs healing unless a soul has become complacent and 'stuck' at a certain level of soul evolution.

Retributive Karma: boomerangs back to punish former actions. In other words, what is done to others comes back with a recognisable connection between cause and effect. Retributive karma is rare and only occurs when a soul refuses to evolve.

Recompense Karma: reward is given for the things that the soul 'got right', or for the sacrifices made to help others.

Redemptive Karma: some souls incarnate to help others or to do something specific for the world. Special needs children may have chosen to come back to help their parents learn a lesson such as compassion and caring. Other souls take on tasks that will help to clear collective karma.

Attitudinal Karma: builds over several lives and arises out of an intransigent attitude, ingrained behaviour or an intractable or habitual emotional stance. It often manifests at the physical level. Mental states such as doubt can also affect the next life. Positive attitudes, such as a loving nature or innate trust, brought forward would creative positive effects in the present life.

Organic Karma: reflects injuries or conditions from other lives. Positive organic karma can arise when the soul has worked hard to strengthen an organ such as the heart in a past life. Organic karma can also arise from soul choices that have caused other people to suffer, and when the soul reincarnates, it has to learn what it feels like to go through that pain or trauma.

The Karmic Treadmill: destructive patterns that have not been outgrown go round and around. The soul is on a karmic treadmill. The expectation is reinforced, and round the soul goes again. Not only that, children will most probably inherit the attitude so that it multiplies.

Karma of Work: what a person did in another life, how they behaved with regard to work, what they experienced, or the skills they possessed, may manifest again in the present life. The karma of work arises from causes such as past behaviour, ethical decisions or choices made. Positive work karma creates skills and vocations in the present life.

Technological Karma: stems from having had to make ethical decisions about the use, or misuse, of technology in the past. It can also apply to having fought against the introduction of new technology – especially when this would have been beneficial to humankind. Technological karma can relate to all periods in history but most often involved industrial and technological revolutions and their effects on modern life. It can also occur with someone who misused or was abused by technology.

Vocational Karma: work is carried over from another incarnation. Vocational karma is an opportunity to capitalise on past skills and abilities.

Symbolic Karma: a present life condition symbolises what was done in the past. It can be a form of allegory.

Communication Karma: how and what was communicated can lead to communication karma. Words have been used to stir revolutions, to revile and condemn people, and to gain power over others. People have passed on gossip and scandal, made or ruined other people's reputations. They have told truths and untruths; been open and honest or secretive and devious.

Ideological Karma: attachment to a belief, no matter how worthy, creates ideological karma. Imposing beliefs on other people also creates this karma. The beliefs may be religious, philosophical or purely secular.

Karma of Hypocrisy: having said one thing, or done things a certain way, and yet believed something totally different gives rise to the karma of hypocrisy. As does a people-pleasing 'anything for a quiet life' approach to life. Hypocrisy arises from a lack of spiritual conviction and inner truth, or a betrayal of truth.

Karma of Mockery: mocking other people's afflictions, thoughts, beliefs or actions gives rise to the karma of mockery. It is based on not valuing the pathway that another person travels.

'Sins of Omission and Commission': the 'things that have been done that ought not to have been done, and the things that have not been done that should have been done'. If a soul always behaved in a certain way, or consistently refused to take action, or to learn a lesson, then the karma comes around and around until the message is understood. Lives can be experienced as 'sinning' or 'sinned against' as the soul struggles to find a way out of the repeating pattern. The soul's failure to take a risk can accrue karma just as strongly as the soul who takes an unwise risk and fails.

Relationship Karma: can operate in families, love affairs, friendships and business relationships. Sometimes a bond of true love unites a couple down through the ages, but this is not always so. Hatred can be the cause of powerful attachments. Some people will not let go of someone they 'love', and have to come back with that person until they can do so. The lesson can be painful, especially when the other person does not recognise the 'love'. Retribution can be a component of relationship karma, as can recompense and reparation. (See *The Soulmate Myth*.)

Pacts and Promises: vows made in another life can strongly affect the present. They may involve another person or be personal.

Phobias: stem from overwhelming fear. They have a karmic root.

Karma-in-suspension: not all karma can be dealt with at once, some of it remains in suspension to be dealt with at some other time – which may or may not occur during the present life depending on how other factors progress.

Karma-in-the-making: what goes on at the present time creates future karma. Each thought, deed, action and belief creates karma for the next life.

The karma of Grace: when sufficient work has been done, or all that is possible has been accomplished, the soul can move on through grace. It can step off the karmic wheel.

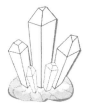

The karmic groove

What goes around may come around, but it never ends up exactly the same place... Like a record on a turntable, all it takes is one groove's difference and the universe can be on into a whole 'nother song.

Thomas Pynchon, *Inherent Vice*

Many people experience karma as an endlessly repeating cycle playing itself out with subtle variations, rather like the film *Groundhog Day*. This is because deeply ingrained, reactive patterns have arisen over many lifetimes. The soul becomes 'stuck in a groove', going over and over the same old ground, unable to move forward freely. So, a soul may become stuck in a feeling of unworthiness for instance – and will attract many situations that, apparently, confirm that unworthiness. It will be attracted to a family in which unworthiness is a transgenerational theme. The soul may look to others for support, seeking worth through their eyes rather than self-validation. The underlying pattern will be reiterated life after life until the soul can break out of the bondage of unworthiness and learn to recognise its own innate worth.

The 'groove-type' pattern frequently happens in relationships where two souls, or whole families, incarnate together again and again, despite the fact that they have long ago learned everything they had to learn from each other, and have repaid any karmic debts they had. They return together from habit – and even hatred can become a pattern. At some point, they have to learn to let go of each other and move on.

There can be a 'swinging pendulum' groove pattern where, in one life, one extreme is lived out and then, in the next, the other extreme. Then back to the first and so on. The pendulum may swing between dominator and dominated, abused and abuser, rebel and conformist, codependent and loner. The soul must find the middle way.

The unfinished business of a relationship is often concerned with one soul taking responsibility for itself. Or, giving up responsibility for someone else, or learning to be independent. Codependence is a common pattern in which the soul feels it will die without the other person. Similar patterns include saviour-rescuer and victim-martyr, or persecutor and persecuted scenarios in which one soul can take the dominant role or the partners can alternate roles. Walking away from the role can be an enormous challenge but may be the only solution to the recurring motif. Unless, of course, karmic and ancestral healing is undertaken. Which is where crystals can intercede.

If you suspect you might be stuck in a karmic groove, take a look at the people around you and the way you interact. Have you been there before? Does it feel like the same old, same old? Do the same situations keep coming up time after time, even if you change partners or job or location? If so, you are in a groove.

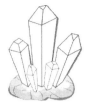

Karmic and ancestral causes of dis-ease

Karmic dis-ease, based on the soul's dis-ease, arises out of wounds, injuries, attitudes and patterns or curses carried forward from past into present via the 'karmic blueprint' and the inherited 'junk DNA' that creates a new body. This dis-ease may be physical, emotional, mental, spiritual or karmic. For example, self-criticism in the past may result in a communication block in the present or could manifest as physical throat problems. It is not a matter of punishment or blame but of balancing out the past and allowing the soul to evolve.

Causes of karmic dis-ease

- Soul unrest
- Soul intention
- Need to develop specific qualities
- Past life repression of pain refuses to be ignored any longer
- Attitudinal karma

- Close-mindedness
- The karmic treadmill
- Bigotry or lack of empathy for others
- Unwillingness to help others
- Organic karma
- Direct carryover of affliction or disability
- Redemptive karma
- Non-development of creative potential
- Conflict from several past life personas
- Strongly negative past life self trying to manifest again, vows
- Curses or ill-wishing

If Healing Does Not Occur

- A soul may not have finished evolving through the condition.
- A soul may be trying to 'get better' for the wrong reasons.
- A soul may be entrenched in 'reparation-restitution' mode.
- A soul may be offering someone else a soul lesson, or an opportunity to change and grow.

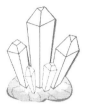

Activating the karmic credit card

As we've seen, not all karma is 'bad karma' and endless reparation is not required. Souls create beneficial karma too, and this can override the most challenging of karmic situations. Switch on your beneficial karma and connect to your soul learning with this simple, high vibration crystal layout.

- *Ground yourself thoroughly.*
- *Lie down comfortably and place a Smoky Elestial Quartz crystal at your feet.*
- *Place a high vibration three-chambered heart crystal such as Petalite or Azeztulite at the base of your breastbone.*
- *Place a Blue Moonstone or other alta major chakra crystal in the hollow at the base of your skull.*
- *Place Blue Kyanite or other appropriate crystal on the alta major chakra and bring the Akashic Record close to you.*
- *Place a Preseli Bluestone or other crystal on your soma chakra.*

- *Place a Trigonic Quartz or other soul crystal point down above your head as high as you can reach.*
- *Gently massage the past life chakras just behind your ears.*
- *Place your hands with fingertips touching just below the three-chambered heart crystal and breathe deeply.*
- *Ask the crystals to download your beneficial karma and soul learning into whichever chakras are appropriate.*
- *Ask that the positive karma will be activated as appropriate and that the people with whom you share the soul learning will make themselves known to you if this is appropriate.*
- *When the download is complete, gather up the crystals in the order that you laid them down. Close the chakras above and around your head.*
- *Ensure that your grounding cord is in place.*

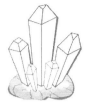

The Akashic Record

The Akashic Record is an ongoing record of the journey of the soul, the evolution of this and other worlds, and the future of All That Is. Anyone living now has probably lived on Earth before – and will live again, possibly on Earth but most definitely in other realms. Fortunately we don't have to understand how the field can exist nor how it works in order to be able to utilise it for healing. While everyone 'sees' the Record in their own way, the underlying experience is the same. It is a connection to what we can call the cosmic memory field.

The Record is not a record of a fixed fate but rather a fluid outline map of a soul's journey with all the potentialities that opens up. It goes way out into the future with myriad possibilities opening up as well as accessing the past. A hologram of all that is and might be, it is not in any one place as it permeates our whole universe. Our souls are connected to this hologram, each carrying a small piece that contains the whole. Incarnated and discarnate souls can visit the Records.

Souls play out the destinies we planned for ourselves

in the space between lives – the interlife – although this plan may be powerfully affected by the karma we have accrued and by soulplans from others' lives that, although outdated, still overlay our soul's intention (see *The Book of Why: Understanding Your Soul's Journey*). Our soulplan may also be sabotaged by transgenerational themes and issues. By accessing the Akashic Record, we can see what we have been (our previous lives), what we might have been (our unlived lives) and what we might be – our potential futures depending on what choices we make. All of which are mapped in the Record.

To use the Record for healing you can visualise it, or use a picture of a tree with deep roots as a symbolic 'Record' on which you place appropriate crystals (see page 278).

Reading the Akashic Record

Do not attempt to read the Record for someone for whom you don't have permission whether from the person themselves or their Higher Self. Once you become practised you can adapt the method to suit yourself and the information you are seeking. When you first begin, you'll probably have 'practice runs'. That is, you'll get glimpses but they may not make much sense. This is rather like tuning one of those old-fashioned television sets in. You get a lot of static and a few glimpses of images that move on quickly before you can fix them in place, and then gradually you can tune into an image, hold it and have the scene move on slowly enough to understand what you are seeing. Because moments of great emotional trauma and soul dramas seem to make the biggest impression on the record, these are what tend to be seen first and it is possible to tune into a specific historical event without actually having been there. If you find a scene distressing, remember that you are seeing it objectively at a distance, not reliving or embodying it. The scene can be reframed into a different outcome if it needs healing. You can also attune to the various potential futures that exist in each. This also works well if you want to assess the outcome of ancestral healing on future generations.

It is useful to have a friend with you when you first try this exercise. Ensure that the friend has been instructed, "Don't try to pull me out suddenly if you think I'm contacting a traumatic scene." "Treat me gently and only intervene if I ask you." (You can arrange a signal such as lifting your arm to indicate you need help.) What is essential is that this companion is apprised of the way to bring you back safely should you wander too far or get lost in a scene:

To guide a return

- *Withdraw your attention from that scene and disconnect your energies and awareness.* Make your way back to the lift, asking your Higher Self to accompany you. Step into the lift and press the button for 'everyday reality'. The lift will bring you down through the vibrations until you reach the place you* *started from. Step out of the lift and be aware of leaving the past (or the future) behind. Cross the meadow until you reach your starting place.*

- *Slowly return your awareness to the room, come into the present moment [if appropriate state the date and time]. Take a few deep breaths and then slowly open your eyes. Wiggle your fingers and toes and make sure your feet make a strong connection to the earth.*
- *Holding a grounding crystal facilitates the return.*

*If there is any hesitancy about returning, your friend should ask if there is any unfinished business that needs attention and then find a creative way to deal with it if there is – higher selves are usually all too willing to offer assistance with this. Tea and a biscuit usually completes the process of return to everyday awareness.

To read the record

- *Settle yourself comfortably in a quiet place where you will not be disturbed. Turn off the phone. Place a grounding crystal at your feet and ensure that your grounding root is in place. Close your eyes. Open your base chakra and let it hold you safely and gently so that you can bring the information down to Earth.*
- *Open the causal vortex chakra and bring it close to you (see page 53).*
- *Breathing rhythmically and easily, withdraw your attention from the outside world. If any thoughts pass through your mind that do not relate to this work, let*

them pass on by. Place a Preseli Bluestone, Chrysotile or other Akashic Record crystal on your third eye (above and between your eyebrows) and allow your inner sight to open.

- *Now see yourself in a beautiful meadow. Feel the ground beneath your feet, smell the air and enjoy being in this beautiful place. Let your feet take you over to a small building that is away to one side.*

- *When you reach the building, open the door and go in. In front of you, you will see a lift with its doors standing open waiting for you. Inside the lift are several buttons. One is marked 'Akashic Records'. Press the button and let the lift take you up through the dimensions to where the Record is housed.*

- *As the lift doors open, your Higher Self steps forward to meet you to conduct you through the multi-media experience that is the Akashic Record. Your Higher Self may take out the Book of your Life for you to read, or hand you a DVD or show computer graphics (most of the Record seems to have been digitalised now). It may show you the many rooms and dimensions of the Record. Simply let the experience unfold before you with your Higher Self guiding the process for your highest good. If you have any specific questions, put them before your Higher Self and ask to be shown the answers as and when appropriate.*

- *When you have completed your Akashic session, disconnect your energies from the scene, thank your Higher Self and ask it to accompany you back to the lift.*

- *Step into the lift and press the button for 'everyday present reality'. The lift will bring you down through the vibrations until you reach the place you started from. Step out of the lift and be aware of leaving the past (or the future) behind. Cross the meadow until you reach your starting place.*
- *Remove the crystal from your third eye. Close your causal vortex shutters.*
- *Slowly return your awareness to the room. Take a few deep breaths and then slowly open your eyes. Move your fingers and toes and make sure your feet make a strong connection to the Earth. Pick up your grounding crystal and hold it for a few moments. Have a drink and a biscuit.*

*If there is any hesitancy about returning, ask your Higher Self if there is unfinished business that needs attention and then find a creative way to deal with it if there is – higher selves are usually willing to offer assistance with this.

Intuiting the Record

Some people never 'see' the Record as vivid pictures but they get bodily sensations and intuitions when performing clearings and readings. If you feel a sensation in any part of your body or an emotion, let it grow and become stronger. Let the feeling tell you the story that lies behind it. Hold one of the past life seeing crystals and say to yourself, "If I knew what the story was it would be…" You'll be surprised how often the answer pops into your awareness. Then let the feeling or sensation go. Or, with the assistance of appropriate crystals, reframe it. Follow up with appropriate crystal healing sessions until the issue is resolved and the necessary reprogramming of the 'junk DNA' and the ancestral line has been completed.

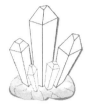

Clearing the timelines

Timelines weave a complex web of intersecting lives: yours and others. When timelines get 'snagged' together, they pull issues or contacts from one life into another in an inappropriate manner. To release the timelines, place appropriate crystals on the illustration wherever you intuit a separation is required. Alternatively, place a crystal on each nexus (joining point). Leave the layout in place and add or remove crystals whenever it feels right to do so. Spray the crystals regularly with Petaltone Clear2Light or Z14, or other crystal cleansing and energizing spray.

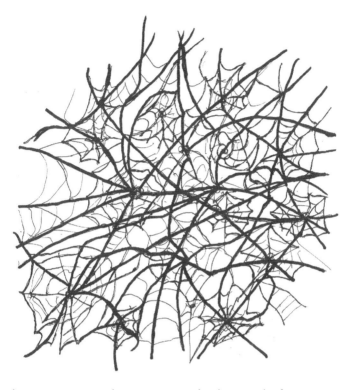

Intersecting timelines against a background of previous lives and different timeframes.

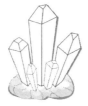

Karmic clearing for the planet

Can we find a way to pull together? A way that unites rather than divides us? Can we share what we know openly and without jealousy, honouring every contribution? Can we be butterflies dancing a new universe into being? After all, if we can't, who can?
Judy Hall, *Earth Blessings*

It is not only people who have karma. The land beneath our feet does too. It stems not only from what has been enacted upon it – the wars, the pogroms, the curses and blessings, and the rape of resources – but also what has been created by the Earth itself – the 'natural disasters' and the consequent devastation. This is another collective area where no one person is responsible, but certain people have incarnated with the redemptive intention of being healers for the planet. One of the simplest ways of earth-healing is to place crystals in the landscape or, failing that, on a map of the area. It is also possible to utilise the Earth's own chakra and meridian grid, and the powerful vortexes within it, placing crystals to support and rebalance the grid. There isn't room to go into the details of earth-healing here, but see *Earth Blessings*.

The Seven Major Earth Chakras

Base: Mount Shasta, California (alternative: Grand Canyon, Sedona Black Mesa, USA)
Sacral: Lake Titicaca, South America (alternative: Machu Picchu, Amazon River)
Solar Plexus: Uluru, Australia
Heart: Glastonbury, England (alternative: River Ganges, India; Dobogoko, Hungary)
Throat: Great Pyramid, Egypt
Third Eye: Kuh-e Malek Siah, Iran (alternative: Mount Fuji, Japan)
Crown: Mount Kailash, Tibet

The elemental vortexes

Four elemental vortexes have also been identified which drive the whole energy grid:

Earth – Table Mountain, Cape Town, South Africa
Air – Great Pyramid–Mount of Olives
Fire – Haleakala Crater, Hawaii
Water – Lake Rotopounamu, North Island, New Zealand

The Earth's crystalline grid

The crystal can still be seen in twelve pentagonal slabs covering the surface of the globe (a dodecahedron as suggested by Socrates who said, "The real Earth viewed from above is supposed to look like one of those balls made of twelve pieces of skin sewn together"), overlaid with twenty equilateral triangles. The entire geometric structure, they claim, can be seen in its influence on the siting of ancient civilisations, on earth faults, magnetic anomalies, and many other otherwise unrelated locations which are placed either at the intersections of the grid, or along its lines.

www.ancient-wisdom.com

In the 1960s, three Russian scientists proposed that the Earth was a giant crystal. In an article published in *Khimiya i Zhizn*, the science journal of the Academy of Sciences, they put forward the theory that a "matrix of cosmic energy" had been built into the structure of the Earth during its formation. This lattice could still be perceived today by those with eyes to see. This concept is extremely useful for karmic healing as crystals placed on the lattice send healing throughout the whole.

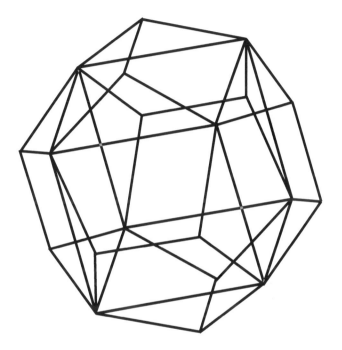

Illustration 7: View of the Earth as a 'Giant Crystal' as
envisioned by a group of three Russian scientists in the
1960s. www.ancient-wisdom.com/theworldgrid.htm

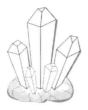

Suitable layouts

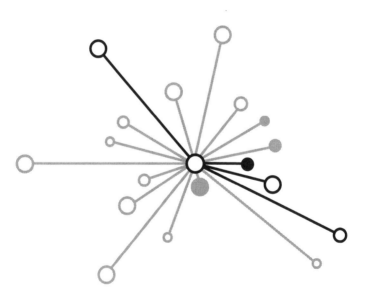

A sunburst layout radiates healing energy into the landscape.
Place as many crystals as are appropriate along each 'arm'
with a central karma clearer in the centre.

A pentangle draws light down into the land to dissolve karma. Place a light-bringing crystal such as Anandalite or Selenite at the topmost point; Earth detoxifying crystals such as Aragonite sputniks or Smoky Quartz at the bottom; and karma clearers on the 'arms'. Join up the points with a crystal wand or the power of your mind.

Practical example

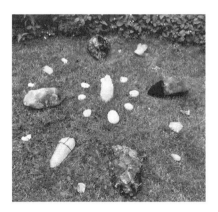

Earth clearing full moon grid on the Dorset Cursus: Smoky and Smoky Elestial Quartz, Selenite and Flint.

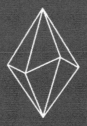

Part III
Soul Retrieval
and Spirit Release

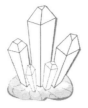

The divided soul

I awoke in the deepest night to find I had been divided from myself. There lay my body sleeping and dreaming, and I was outside it; awakening. When we dream we may take shapes other than our own; a man may be his brother, a woman a king, and never question it. So, with the certainty born of a dream, I knew I'd become my own shadow.
Sarah Micklem, *Firethorn*

I've been using crystals to facilitate spirit release and soul retrieval for over 45 years. Whilst I believe that these activities are best carried out by trained specialists, there are times when you may suddenly be confronted with the need to retrieve lost soul parts or release attachments. Emergency action has to be taken there and then. This is where crystals come in, especially when supported by purpose-made essences. I find these gentle, compassionate tools invaluable for three reasons:

- They protect my own energies, creating an objective interface at which I can work safely. The crystal stands at the border between my personal energy field, the other person and the soul part or attachment, creating a barrier so that nothing can attach to me. Crystals also maintain a sacred and energetically clean space in which to work.

- Crystals energetically heal and purify a soul part that is returning. They facilitate release and call in higher helpers and divine light to move a spirit on, facilitating the work. Crystals can, when needed, provide a 'home' for a spirit or entity until it can be moved on or returned to whence it came. They also act rather like a net to hold anything undesirable until it can be moved on to an appropriate place, rather than setting it free to attach to another vulnerable soul.
- Crystals energetically integrate the soul part back into the auric field, or seal the site of an attachment once it has been cleared, purifying and healing the aura, object or environment so that nothing else can attach.

So, what do I mean by soul retrieval and spirit release?

Soul loss, soul splits and soul fragmentation

It may surprise you to learn that souls are not 'all of a piece'. Part of the soul, the Higher Self, remains less deeply incarnated than the rest and can, therefore, have a much wider view of the purpose, potential and outcome of an incarnation. But souls can also fragment. Soul loss, sometimes known as a soul split or fragmentation, is a condition that leaves you particularly vulnerable to psychic attack and to spirit attachment as it creates a vacuum in the auric field. Souls can split, combine and recombine with other members of an overall soul group, for instance. Parts of the soul can detach at moments of trauma, high drama, or even at points of extreme joy. They may remain in a previous life, especially if there has been a traumatic death or if a body has not been given appropriate burial rites. But souls can also split into two or more pieces and appear to be totally different entities.

It is not uncommon to find that a soul has parts in different physical incarnations at the same time. Soul loss almost invariably accompanies post-traumatic stress disorder (PTSD). Thinking of the soul as a hologram helps in understanding this process. A hologram can be both here and there, split and yet still cohesive. Soul retrieval, bringing together and reintegrating lost soul parts, helps you to feel centred, balanced and whole once more. Experiencing the light carried by the crystal penetrating every cell of your being, at all levels, not only returns your soul to your body but also helps to heal the repercussions of soul loss in the 'junk-DNA' and karmic etheric body.

Gathering up pieces of the soul so that it can reintegrate has been practised by shamans and soul retrieval practitioners throughout aeons of time. It may be extremely helpful in cases where someone is not fully present or in certain psychiatric illnesses. Pieces of a soul may be left earlier in the present life, or in other lives, and it is part of soul retrieval and past life therapy practice to retrieve and reintegrate these fragments as appropriate. Bringing them back through a crystal purifies, heals and re-energizes the soul fragment. However, there are times when reintegrating a soul part is not appropriate, in which case a crystal can act as a container for that soul until it becomes apparent where to direct the soul or putting it into the care of the Higher Self.

Soul loss

Parts of the overall self may remain at past life deaths, traumatic or joyful moments and so on rather than incarnate with the main soul at birth into the present life. Soul loss may also occur during the current life.

A soul split over two lives

Soul loss can also occur when a past life or ancestral persona breaks through and is acted out. Especially if the soul part left in the previous incarnation is still extremely active. We've seen how timelines can intertwine and interweave. Sometimes the barrier between two timeframes thins to the point where one can intrude into the other. In extreme cases, this can feel as though two people are inhabiting the same skin, or that you have been taken over by someone else. In *The Book of Why* I quoted the case of Donovan, a Vietnam vet. He was a soul who had a 'foot in both camps'. Although Donovan was apparently living in a present life as an alienated outsider (itself a symptom of soul loss and past life persona break-through), he was also concurrently living a life as a soldier in the Vietnam war. That life had broken through in spontaneous regression, but in the previous life, he had also taken a huge amount of drugs which facilitated the time travelling. His soul was split between the two lives and there was a huge crossover so that Donovan didn't really know where he belonged. He couldn't function properly in his 'present' life because so much of him was 'back there' stuck in a life that was cut short – and so much of 'back there' was operating in his current life.

Donovan's vivid dreams, recollections and intuitions tried to take him to a point where his soul could reinte-grate and heal the past. Had he had a therapist facili-tating this, it could have been quicker – and smoother – but 'doing it himself' was a part of the alienated outsider persona he'd carried over, and he needed to reach the insights himself. It was a part of his soul intention.

There are many people walking around in a similar fogged, fragmented and disconnected state as a past life persona has taken over part, or all, of their present life personality. Soul fragmentation leaves such people open to psychic attack or attachment from 'lost', 'stuck' or 'alien' souls and such like. Complex soul release, reintegration or past life healing may be required in addition to soul retrieval. This really is a job for an expert (see Resources and page 214 for how to move a stuck soul on in an emergency).

Subtle soul splits

Widely differing past life experiences may create a subtle soul split within an incarnated soul who is apparently all of a piece but is actually experiencing an inner split within the same lifetime. The sexuality-spirituality axis split is common and powerfully affects the ability to be intimate in the present life, or to form a parental or other bond. If someone has taken a vow of celibacy in a previous life, for instance, and not rescinded it, it may be re-enacted through a subconscious past life memory borne deep in the soul. The person will feel guilty during a sexual act. But equally, another part of the soul, which has enjoyed sexual engagements in the past, may be pushed to the fore as a reaction against the celibacy. The two personas will battle it out, one appearing uppermost and then the other. Similarly, an ancestor can intrude in something that is stronger than a light spirit attachment. This is particularly so when the ancestor has a vested interest, or unfinished agenda, in certain situations coming to fruition. In such cases, the 'ancestor' may be an earlier incarnation of the same soul.

Sometimes, however, a soul 'splits' and comes into incarnation in two distinctly separate bodies. This is generally because 'one half' incarnates to assist or facilitate the 'other half' in a specific task. Nevertheless, soul splits can occur for more traumatic, less deliberately planned, reasons. Some 'splits' reintegrate after death, but others continue as separate souls and cannot be reintegrated during the present lifetime. These types of soul splits may need the assistance of expert help, but the symptoms and first aid treatment are the same.

Crystals help to purify the soul part and to reintegrate it. Calling the soul home, whether it's a split-off child part, an earlier past life part that hasn't incarnated, or the result of trauma or abuse in the present life, is facilitated with either a Brandenberg or Spirit Quartz, but Fulgarite was traditionally used by American shamans to collect the soul part and blow it back into the heart.

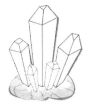

Signs of soul loss, soul split, or past life or ancestral persona breakthrough

The immediate symptoms of soul loss or the break-through of a past life or ancestral persona – which has a similar effect – can be interchangeable with spirit attachment signals (see page 208) but there are additional subtle signals that may take more time to be recognised:

- Feeling vague, nebulous and insubstantial. Somehow 'not there'. To an outside eye, incomplete and fragmented.
- Feeling like a different person after a shock or traumatic life event.
- Multiple selves try to make themselves known, with sudden switches and memory loss.
- Problems with time.
- 'Blank' eyes stare into the distance.
- No eye contact.
- 'Someone else' looks out from the eyes.
- A profound sense of disconnection from everyday

life.

- Behaviour is out of character with normal persona.
- Obsessive, escapist or addictive behaviour including sexual.
- Constant 'busyness', never rests.
- Severe insomnia.
- Constant fears and anxieties.
- Unusual thought patterns, sometimes self-destructive.
- Intense dreams or fantasies with a nightmarish quality.
- Hearing voices.
- A feeling of being controlled by someone else.
- Sudden overwhelming bouts of tiredness or yawning and chronic fatigue.
- Overwhelming sugar cravings.
- Memories of portions of life especially shock or trauma have been blocked out.
- Prolonged periods of depression.
- PTSD
- Everyone is kept at arm's length, no openness even to close friends or family.
- A profound numbness invades every part of life. Issues are not recognised or dealt with.
- Psychosomatic dis-eases are present.
- Severe disappointment in life.
- A deep sense of unworthiness prevails.
- A 'dark night of the soul' is constantly undergone.
- There is no sense of purpose or meaning in life.

- Things are done because they have to be done. There is no joy or purpose in it.
- Overexcitement, constantly 'revved up'.
- Being on a constant emotional or mental 'high'.
- Rapid, constant and somewhat random chatter.
- Longing for an authentic self.

Healing a soul split and returning a soul fragment

This layout calls home and integrates soul fragments that are ready to return. It is also suitable for healing a soul split, but healing a soul split in this way is only applicable when both parts of the soul are contained within a single incarnated human being – even though the two parts of the soul may be acting as though they are separate individuals; or when one part is in incarnation and the other is not. It is not suitable for cases where two different physical bodies are involved (that has to wait until at least one has passed beyond death of the physical body). Calling on the Higher Self (the part of the soul not fully in physical incarnation) to assist facilitates the process. Dowse to ascertain which would be the best crystals for you. Have a Selenite crystal to hand in case you need a container for a soul fragment that is not yet ready to reintegrate. In this exercise there is nothing to do, simply allow the process to take place.

Higher Self

The 'Higher Self' is the part of ourself that is not fully in incarnation as it vibrates at a higher rate, and, therefore, has a much clearer picture of why we are here and where we are going. It carries the memory of our previous lives, our soulplan – and our soul overlays and soul splits. It constantly monitors the whole of the soul, whether fragmented or not. The Higher Self acts as guide, mentor and information assistant to the soul in incarnation. It is a useful guide to facilitate soul retrieval.

Self-help soul retrieval exercise

- *Cleanse and balance your chakras as far as possible (see page 56).*
- *Ensure that your grounding root is in place.*
- *Ensure that you are in a quiet, protected space.*
- *Place a Trigonic Quartz, Shiva Shell, Preseli Bluestone or other soul retrieval crystal on your soma chakra (mid-hairline just above the third eye).*
- *Place an Anandalite, Trigonic or other soul retrieval crystal on your heart seed chakra (base of your breastbone below the heart chakra).*
- *With the fingers of each hand, tap either side of your breastbone, about a hand's breath below your collarbone on the 'spirit ground' points on the illustration below. If*

it feels appropriate you can also tap these points, the 'sore spots' and the 'baggage points' with a small Trigonic, Brandenberg or Lemurian Seed crystal.

- *Ask your Higher Self to call back to you any soul fragments that are ready to return, or to repair a split soul if this is appropriate. Request your Higher Self to ensure that only fragments that rightfully belong with your soul at the present moment will return to you.*
- *The soul fragments will pass through the crystals to purify and re-energize them as they reintegrate, leaving the past behind them but bringing forward any wisdom learned.*
- *As the soul part returns, absorb it along with the crystal energy into every cell of your body and at all energetic levels. Feel the light carried in the crystal healing and reintegrating your whole being.*
- *If a soul portion is not yet ready to reintegrate, place it in the Selenite crystal. When the exercise is complete, ask if it is more appropriate to send that soul part to the care of the Higher Self for the time being. If so, ask the crystal to release the soul part into the care of your Higher Self. If it prefers to remain in the crystal for the time being, check out every few days what the appropriate action is for that soul part. It may be that it stays with the Higher Self for the duration of the current life.*
- *When the integration is complete, pass Anandalite or Selenite round your whole aura to heal and seal it once again.*

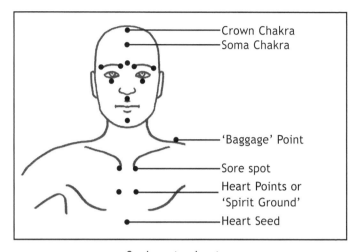

Soul retrieval points

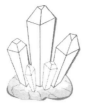

Spirit attachment

In spirit attachment, a soul or spirit, a thought form (see page 45), or an entity from outside our universe, is attached to, or overly influences, a body to which it does not belong. Spirit attachment can only occur where there is an auric or chakra weakness, so, in addition to releasing the attachment, it is only sensible to take good care of your chakras, giving them a regular cleanse (see page 56 and Chakra attachments on page 62). The symptoms of spirit attachment, perhaps not surprisingly, are extremely close to those of soul loss (see page 201).

When releasing a spirit, appropriate, cleansed crystals can either be put directly on to the body, spiralled over the chakras or placed in a grid around the room, in the environment or around the physical body. The crystal, which carries unconditional love, acts as a psychopomp conducting the soul through the spirit world and other dimensions to its appropriate 'home' for the next stage of its journey. Crystals for release work well placed in the aura about a foot out from the physical body as that is where many of the more subtle attachments occur. Sweeping the whole aura with an appropriate crystal often clears minor attachments without needing to know the full story and will send a spirit to the light, dissolve a thought form, or detach undue influence. A crystal with a point will pull out energies or ties when pointed towards and then spiralled away from the body, and draw in light when pointed towards it once again. Crystals need to be cleansed before and after spirit release work or healing. Always ask that a crystal will work for the highest good of all and that a spirit or an entity will be returned to its rightful and appropriate place in whatever dimension or timeframe that may be.

Signals that a spirit may be attached

- When you look in the mirror you do not recognise yourself looking back.
- You feel that you have lost a part of yourself and gained something *other*.
- You feel as though there are multiple persons within you.
- You feel as though you have become a different person after a severe shock or traumatic life event.
- You feel as though you are not in control. You hear commands from voices that are not your own.
- You experience obsessions and addictions quite suddenly, out of the blue, and especially after a traumatic experience.

See also the Signs of soul loss page 201.

However, it is sensible to bear in mind that the signals

that suggest attachment may also be symptoms of a psychiatric illness or mental breakdown. Lost and malicious spirits are attracted to someone who has no defences against them, so the more depressed or psychiatrically disturbed a person is, the more likely it is that there could be an attachment present. But equally, having an attachment can lead to mental or physical dis-ease. Over-medication or addiction to certain drugs, whether legally prescribed or not, can also lead to spirit attachment and (additional) psychiatric disturbance.

Spirit attachment can be seen in the eyes, which are blank with 'no one home' or 'someone else' looks out from them. The attaching spirit usually seeks to experience something it was addicted to in life or to control someone. It may be simply lost or be malicious. Attachments are not confined to human beings and may arise from thought forms or alien sources. It's not always an external attachment *although it may feel like it is*. It may equally well be projection/repressed qualities/obsessive thoughts manifesting apparently externally. Spirit may also be attached to an object rather than a person. It is sensible to bear in mind that not all attaching spirits will have left their physical body. The living can 'possess' or overly influence the living. Attachments can arise from the thoughts and feelings of others who try to influence or control, or who try to clutch on to your strength – a very common experience for healers, readers and counsellors. It's as though they have their hooks into you (see below).

Spirit attachment definition

Spirit attachment means that a discarnate – or possibly part of an incarnate – spirit or entity has entered a living person's energy field, and is influencing it. Or, that it has become attached to a place. It can only occur when an energy field is weak and depleted, and when someone does not fully inhabit their body and their soul is not fully present so there is a 'gap' or vacuum in the auric field. It often arises out of momentary loss of energetic boundaries such as in shock or trauma, drink or drug taking, or the effects of anaesthetic. It is common in cases of depression or debilitating illnesses like ME. But it may also stem back to other lives or deliberate psychic attack.

---

210   Some lost souls may be deeply troubled and their interaction with the living can be malicious. They may have unfinished business, or powerful desires especially for control over another person or to re-experience substance abuse. Other souls are suspended and simply do not know how to move on or to let go. Sometimes they do not even know that they are dead – after all, they feel very much alive! They may wonder why everyone around them appears to ignore them – and some do all they can to gain attention. Other souls are simply clinging to what they know and, therefore, attach to remain earthbound.

This is work for an experienced therapist but if you do become involved, wherever possible, ask for family and friends, or a guide or mentor, to meet the spirit being released to take it home.

Types of earthbound spirits

- **Ghosts:** more like photographic imprints left behind than actual spirits. They can be recognised by their lack of awareness, repetition of actions and general opacity.
- **Those who are frightened to leave:** further progress is blocked because of fear of the unknown or expectation of punishment for deeds on Earth.
- **Those with unfinished business:** in addition to a desire for revenge, incomplete endings, soul agendas or contracts that were not completed may hold a soul back, as may a body from a former life that did not receive the appropriate burial rights. The spirit remains with the previous life body, or attaches to the person with whom there is unfinished business.
- **Those who are disorientated and confused:** the spirit is not aware of being dead. The passing has been sudden and traumatic. The moment to leave was missed. The spirit is still trying to get attention on the Earth plane and is unaware of assistance waiting on the astral or etheric plane.
- **Those who want to stay to fulfil a craving:** the spirit has addictions which can, seemingly, be

fulfilled by taking over another physical body so the spirit stays close to the Earth plane. The addiction may be substance related or person-centred.

- **Malicious:** mischievous or vicious, this spirit has an intention to cause trouble or seek revenge.
- **Thought forms:** beings that have not had an independent existence but rather have been created by a mind or idea.
- **Guardian being:** some spirits remain as a family mentor or spirit of place guardian, such as found at a sacred site. This type of spirit may have outlasted its original purpose. It is always wise to check before moving such a soul on that release is appropriate.

Lost souls and stuck spirits

If an attaching spirit has simply lost the way home, holding one of the spirit release crystals in the Directory (see page 374) and asking that the spirit be taken to the light by his or her guardian angel or attending family members works well, particularly if you light a candle and ask for deceased family members to assist. Petaltone Astral Clear or Clear Tone essences on a Quartz, Brandenberg or Smoky Spirit Quartz crystal, or a programmed Aventurine or Candle Quartz facilitates the process. (Petaltone also includes a specialised release essence available only to practitioners, www.petaltone .co.uk.)

If you are able to communicate with the spirit – placing a Yellow Labradorite (Bytownite) or Apophyllite pyramid on your third eye facilitates this – ask if there is anything you can do to assist, what he or she wants. The requests are usually simple and easy to arrange, and often relate to unfinished business. Once you have agreed to do or offer whatever is required or assisted the spirit to do so on the etheric, the spirit moves on helped by the energies of the crystal. If the spirit is deeply entrenched, or is still of the opinion that their advice and assistance is crucial for the well-being of someone still on Earth, then it may take further negotiating by a more experienced practitioner. In which case, leave an energetic net holding the spirit until professional assistance can be found.

The crystal portal

Place a Stibnite crystal crossways over a long-pointed Chlorite Quartz and top with a Selenite wand. This one-way portal soaks up any negativity, releases the soul or attachment and sends it out of the Earth plane and into the Light where it can be handled by wise mentors and soul-rescuers. It is particularly useful for blocking re-entry by spirits.

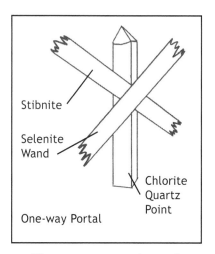

The one-way crystal portal

Emergency Crystal Healing for Spirit Attachment

As the attaching spirit is, usually, an uninvited guest and the influence unsought, I believe this is one occasion when it is not necessary to request the other person's permission to assist them as the spirit is breaching their autonomy and right to choice. If the person is not present, you can either use a photograph or imagine them in the room with you, or use yourself as a surrogate by performing the healing on your own body.

- *As soon as you begin, picture throwing out an energetic net to trap the attaching spirit so that it cannot slip away. This can be a net of light or something stronger like a thick rope cargo net. You can also lay out a crystal net before you start using Selenite, Bronzite or Black*

Tourmaline.

- *Ground yourself thoroughly (see page 19) and place a grounding crystal at your feet. Wear Labradorite or Healer's Gold as a shield.*
- *Open your third eye with Golden Labradorite, Apophyllite or other third eye stone.*
- *Lay a protective Selenite or Black Tourmaline pentangle (five pointed star) on which you have sprinkled Petaltone Astral Clear, Z14 or Clear2Light around you. Join up the points with a crystal wand or the power of your mind. If the person is present, lay Selenite around them.*
- *Light a candle for the spirit to guide the way to the light.*
- *Holding a Brandenberg or Smoky Amethyst (or other crystal from the list), place a Bytownite or Apophyllite on your third eye or on the person with the attaching spirit. Ask that the spirit will make itself known and tell you why it has chosen to stay close to the Earth. Ascertain whether the spirit knows it has passed to another plane of being.*
- *Talk to the spirit as appropriate, addressing his or her concerns and offering unconditional love, reassurance and understanding. Then ask if the spirit is ready to move into the light for healing.*
- *Place appropriate crystals over the soma (mid-hairline), heart and solar plexus chakras. Visualise hands reaching down to help the spirit move into the light. If the spirit is reluctant, ask that his or her guardian angel and Higher Self will assist the process.**

- *Ask if the person who had the attachment needs to call any part of his or her own energy or soul back. If so, call it back with the Brandenberg or Selenite letting it pass through that crystal for purification, and place it over the heart seed. Allow that energy to be reabsorbed.*
- *Now take the Brandenberg or Selenite all the way around the body, sides, front and back, to heal and seal the biomagnetic field.*
- *When the process is complete, detach your contact and close your third eye with a grounding stone. Check that your grounding is still in place.*

[Extracted from *Good Vibrations* with amendments.]

If the attachment is an entity from another dimension you may need to take additional steps, calling on the Galactic Council to call the entity back and placing the crystal portal (see page 213) to close the possibility of any return to this dimension. This is specialised work and should not be attempted unless you are experienced in this type of work. Crystals to assist can be found in the A–Z Directory under 'Spirit release'.

Chakra attachments

Bear in mind that attachments can occur through the chakras and that crystals can be used to 'clean out the hooks'. It's not only discarnate spirits that can attach here. Anyone you have ever had sex with can have left some of their energy field in your lower chakras, for instance. But strong thoughts of lust can lodge there even if there has been no physical contact. You will find emotional attachment hooks in the sacral and solar plexus, thought forms in the third eye, ancestral hooks in the soma or higher chakras and so on. *See Chakra attachments on page 62.*

Spirit attachment to objects

It is not just people and places that can have spirits attached, objects can too – particularly where these have had a cultic value. This is why it is always advisable to cleanse previously-owned jewellery, which may still have a spirit part sentimentally attached. Statues, fetishes and other objects may have a guardian spirit who may need to be released. Less tangible things too can be 'guarded'.

When I was working on the manuscript of *Good Vibrations* it became energetically rather like walking through treacle – heavy and sticky. I actually 'blanked out' for a couple of hours when checking the proofs: classic indications that all was not well. When I checked, the information in that book had a guardian spirit attached whose job it was to keep the esoteric secret. When it was explained to him that things had moved on from his time, that people generally were much more psychically open and aware, and just how badly a book such as that was needed at this time, he agreed to work with us on getting the book out rather than frustrating its progress. He even offered one or two missing pieces. The book benefited from the way he was able to look back at how different things were when he passed to spirit and how such information could have been misused, and then to the present time when it can bring about an enormous energy shift in everyone regardless of their race, creed or lack of metaphysical training. He then moved on to the light of his own accord. I am grateful to him for his assistance.

To cleanse jewellery or cultic objects

You will need:

Faden Quartz or other crystal (see Directory)
Petaltone Astral Clear

- *Ground yourself thoroughly.*
- *Light a candle for the spirit.*
- *Place a drop of Petaltone Astral Clear or other essence on the crystal, place it over or beside the object and ask that the spirit will be taken to the light.*
- *If the object is a gem or crystal, clear and recharge before wearing (see The Basics).*

If the object is a statue or other cultic object, see Moving on a guardian spirit on the following page.

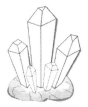

Moving on a guardian spirit

Guardian spirits may relate to a family or to a place. They may or may not have lived on Earth before. They may or may not take humanoid form. Some will have held that role for aeons of time. As attitudes change, and time moves on, their role may become redundant or outdated. But others, particularly at a sacred site or in an ancient landscape, may still have a part to play. Care needs to be taken to ascertain whether or not it is appropriate to move such a spirit on.

To move on a guardian spirit

- *Ground yourself thoroughly (see page 19) and place a grounding crystal at your feet. Wear Labradorite or Healer's Gold as a shield.*
- *Open your third eye with Golden Labradorite, Apophyllite or other third eye stone.*
- *Where possible light a candle for the spirit.*
- *Ask the guardian spirit to make itself known to you.*
- *Establish communication with the spirit wherever possible to ascertain its feelings on the matter. If the guardianship is inappropriate, but that fact is not recog-*

219

nised by the spirit, skilful negotiation may be needed.

- *Thank the spirit for the work it has been doing. Gratitude always assists the process of release.*
- *Ask the spirit if it is ready to relinquish its task and move on. If it is, that may be all that is needed.*
- *If not, and the guardianship really is inappropriate, throw an etheric net over the spirit. Ask that mentors and soul rescuers from the spirit world come to take the guardian to the light. Hold a Selenite wand or other appropriate crystal to assist the process. If necessary, use the Stibnite portal on page 213 to shut off return.*
- *Where necessary, request that a new and appropriate guardian spirit takes over the role. Aragonite or Rhodozite crystals assist a new guardian spirit to settle into land.*
- *When the process is complete, detach your contact and close your third eye with a grounding stone. Check that your grounding is still in place.*

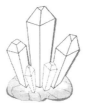

P.S. A Word on Addictions

In the A–Z Directory you will find crystals for specific and general addictions. Many addictions and obsessions arise from soul loss or traumatic events in past lives, previous life experiences, or failed initiation attempts in other lives. In his book *Return from Tomorrow*, Dr George Ritchie documents how, during the Second World War, he died and was placed in the morgue. A 'being of light' took him on a tour of the Afterlife, ranging far and wide. But not everything occurred far from Earth. He was taken to a bar on the Earth plane where sailors drank. All around them he could see the spirits that had passed over addicted to drink. They had been drawn back to what they most craved. As the sailors became drunker, so the spirits slipped into their body to partake of their second-hand fix. Not all of them departed when sobriety returned.

When healing addictions, the cause needs to be located, released and the 'hole' sealed. Detox crystals will be needed and then crystals to support recovery. However, it is wise to remember that, although an attaching spirit may be involved, most addictions also have a karmic or genetic basis and the person must be ready to overcome the addiction themselves. You cannot do it for them. As Michael Vincent so eloquently put it:

I have known for many years now that no matter how many good people line up to help me their time is wasted if I have no wish to help myself.
Michael Vincent, *On Being Alive*

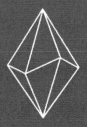

Part IV
Ancestral Healing

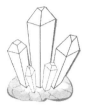

Our ancestors within us

The deeds of an ancestor can create family karma that continues to influence the fate of the family's descendents until the karma is dissolved.
Dr Hiroshi Motoyama

The ancestors are always with us. In some cultures they are honoured, but much of the modern world has lost touch.

Transgenerational issues

Genealogical karma offers a unique opportunity to learn lessons associated with the previous experiences of your loved ones and ancestors, as well as the predecessors of your community, organization, or nation. This level of karma is often very impersonal, and it is farther reaching than the karma of an individual. Healing and resolving family-level and group causal patterns has a liberating effect among all members of the target population. Some experiences are so universal that each person incarnated shares in this inherited karma.
Nicholas Pearson

As Nicholas Pearson points out, genealogical karma goes far beyond the family, and it can incorporate ubiquitous family myths that cross cultures and belief systems. In addition to genetic memory, ancestral memory plays its part in transmitting transgenerational issues. Anything that is spoken about in the family, passing down the ancestral line, becomes 'true' even when it isn't factually correct. But it symbolises the family saga: the myth that is lived by. Family 'memories' of being Russian or other displaced aristocracy, of being swindled out of money or land, or dispossessed from a homeland are common-place. These myths and sagas incorporate themes and issues that may need to be healed not only at the personal level but also on behalf of the greater whole – when one shifts, everything shifts. Common themes often include both extremes of a spectrum, played out in alternate lives or by different members of the family:

Challenging ancestral and transgenerational themes and issues

- Displacement from land of origin
- Power – economic and personal
- Codependence vs. Solitary loner
- Victim-martyr-saviour-rescuer
- Unworthiness, Shame, Guilt, Fear
- Resentment, Criticism
- Abandonment, Rejection
- Family scapegoat
- Bondage

- Submission – 'always comply'
- Rebellion – 'never comply'
- Freedom of the individual, Suppression of the individual
- Perfectionism
- Dominance, Abuse, Addiction
- Aggression (the 'war gene')
- Suppression of emotion
- Disappointment
- 'It's not safe', 'Don't trust…'
- 'Look up to those above us on the social scale'
- 'Know your place', 'Obey those who rule'
- 'We have every right', 'We have no right'
- 'There will never be enough', 'It will be taken away'
- 'It should be different'
- 'In the past we were', 'We were swindled'
- 'People like us don't'

You can probably add your own experience to this list. I've intentionally listed the challenging aspects because these are – generally – what need to be healed and transformed. But it is wise to remember that ancestral themes can also be positive, and once the negative has been released, it creates room for the positive potential to manifest. However, ancestral imperatives such as service to one's country, to one's family, or to one's fellow human beings can have either a positive or challenging effect according to how they played out through the generations – and how much they stifle or thwart an individual's soulplan and soul expansion. This is especially so where such imperatives have become deeply rooted to the exclusion of all else and so a lineage breaker will incarnate to break the pattern.

Family inheritance and DNA

Research into the effects of the ancestors on genetic inheritance has been going on since the early 1960s. Early researchers used isolation tanks and pharmacological triggers to access deep DNA memories and transgenerational experiences. It was postulated that family history, and a carry-over of memories, may have a profound effect on well-being, the effects of earlier experiences subtly altering the family DNA through biological memory amendments. From current scientific investigations, such changes are recorded in the so-called 'junk-DNA' helix (see page 83), negative experiences leading to 'taboo' areas of life or vulnerability to specific dis-eases that pass down the family line. However, positive experiences can imprint useful survival skills and soul qualities:

Over sixty-five years ago the Jewish people were liberated from Nazi Europe. Since that time, researchers have found that the Holocaust has had a psychological, social, and cultural effect on first and second generation survivors… The third generation appears to be reconstructing their grandparents' history, resurfacing their legacy, and in doing so they are realizing the strength and heroic battles their grandparents fought in order to get to the place they are today. Findings indicate that rather than ruminating on the pain of their ancestors, focusing attention on their strength may result in the ability to move past the pathological symptom.

The research suggests that 'epigenetic inheritance', where a person's life experiences can affect the genes of their offspring, may play a huge part in a child's development. While it is widely acknowledged among scientists that DNA does not change, chemical tags that originate from a person's lifestyle and habits can become attached to DNA leading to small differences.

Melissa Kahane-Nissenbaum[14]

*According to the new insights of behavioral epigenetics, traumatic experiences in our past, or in our recent ancestors' past, leave molecular scars adhering to our DNA. Jews whose great-grandparents were chased from their Russian shtetls; Chinese whose grandparents lived through the ravages of the Cultural Revolution; young immigrants from Africa whose parents survived massacres; adults of every ethnicity who grew up with alcoholic or abusive parents – all carry with them more than just memories. Like silt deposited on the cogs of a finely tuned machine after the seawater of a tsunami recedes, **our experiences, and those of our forebears, are never gone, even if they have been forgotten.** They become a part of us, a molecular residue holding fast to our genetic* *scaffolding. The DNA remains the same, but psychological and behavioral tendencies are inherited. You might have inherited not just your grandmother's knobby knees, but also her predisposition toward depression caused by the neglect she suffered as a newborn. Or not. If your grandmother was adopted by nurturing parents, you might be enjoying the boost she received thanks to their love and support. The mechanisms of behavioral epigenetics underlie not only deficits and weaknesses but strengths and resiliencies, too. And for those unlucky enough to descend from miserable or withholding grandparents, emerging drug treatments could reset not just mood, but the epigenetic changes themselves. Like grandmother's vintage dress, you could wear it or have it altered.* **The genome has long been known as the blueprint of life, but the epigenome is life's Etch A Sketch: Shake it hard enough, and you can wipe clean the family curse**... *Just because certain genes have been switched on or off due to our ancestors' experiences does not mean they have to stay turned on or off... We are all the authors of our own lives, but if we do nothing to change the default script that is being played out then the 'broken record' will just keep playing.*[15]

So, the effect of trauma can be reversed, and may well lead to incorporating new strengths and soul learnings into the ancestral line, facilitating evolution. A process that may have commenced fifty, five hundred, five thousand or fifty thousand years ago. However, the drug-based therapy suggested above may not be required as crystals could do the switching for you.

The fears of the fathers

In an experiment carried out at the Emory University School of Medicine, in Atlanta, mice were subjected to fear around the smell of cherry blossom. That fear passed to subsequent generations through amended sperm. So, the previous experience of an ancestor, in addition to personal previous life experience, may underlie seemingly irrational phobias.[16] In commenting on the findings, Dr Brian Dias, from the department of psychiatry at Emory University, said: "We have begun to explore an underappreciated influence on adult behaviour – ancestral experience before conception. From a translational perspective, our results allow us to appreciate how the experiences of a parent, before even conceiving offspring, markedly influence both structure and function in the nervous system of subsequent generations. Such a phenomenon may contribute to the etiology and potential transgenerational transmission of risk for neuropsychiatric disorders such as phobias, anxiety and post-traumatic stress disorder."

The effect of the personal karmic past

When genetic memory is married to a person's own karmic experience, the genetic sequence is switched on. If it does not match the karmic experience, it is less likely to be activated. Of two siblings in a family line that carries alcoholic addiction, for example, one may bypass the addiction but could perhaps display another kind of obsession or compulsive behaviour, while the other becomes a full-blown addict. Similarly, a genetic precondition such as Huntington's Chorea may be triggered, or not, according to personal past life inheritance and the soulplan for the present life.

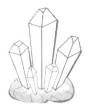

Reading the Ancestral Record

The Akashic Record can be a useful source of insight if you are trying to track the root of a particular issue or attitude. If you are aware of an ancestor with the issue, make that your starting point. If not, ask to be shown the core person who created the genetic memory. (See page 178 for detailed instructions on how to read the Akashic Record.)

To read the Record for an ancestor

Before you read the record for an ancestor:

- *Ask permission and that you will be able to access only what is for the highest good of the transgenerational line.*
- *Ask their Higher Self to assist.*
- *Examine your motives in offering to read, ensure that you are not simply trying to confirm something you have suspected or that the ancestor believed. Don't get caught up in hidden agendas, your own or another person's.*
- *Protect your spleen chakra with an appropriate crystal when reading for someone else. (The spleen chakra is*

located under your left arm about a hand's breadth down.)

- *Open your causal vortex chakra with Blue Kyanite (see page 53) and ground yourself (see page 19) so that energy can flow through.*
- *Ask to be shown the part of the Record that relates to the ancestor or ancestral issue you are dealing with.*
- *Examine that ancestor's life and probable causes. Go back even further if this is not the source.*
- *Look at the potential for reframing and healing any trauma or completing unfinished business from that life. Place appropriate crystals on a photograph or the name of the ancestor, or on a family tree (see pages 236 and 237).*

Healing with far memory photographs

An excellent way of reading ancestral past lives is through the use of photographs. These can be of ancestors living or dead (but remember to ask permission from the Higher Self). It is useful to look at the lives of successive generations. You may be able to identify themes such as scapegoat, sabotage, power, displacement, loss and so on, and take appropriate healing action. You may also be able to identify positive traits that can be activated to replace them.

- *Hold an accessing past lives crystal in one hand.*
- *Holding the photograph in your other hand spend a few moments gazing at it.*
- *Ask your Higher Self to assist the reading.*
- *Ask your Higher Self to connect to the other person's*

Higher Self.

- *Let your eyes go out of focus and continue to gaze at the photo.*
- *The face will go fuzzy and you may see another face or figure superimpose itself. Note how the new person is dressed and how they look. Ask what century they are from and listen for the answer.*
- *Ask to be shown the appropriate past lives. These may appear on the photograph. If not, close your eyes and picture a screen inside your head or just in front of your third eye on which they will be projected. You may also need to speak, without worrying what will come out of your mouth, or to write spontaneously… Do not judge what you hear or see, accept it dispassionately…*
- *When the seeing is complete, turn the photograph face down to disconnect and ask the higher selves to disconnect themselves. Disconnect yourself by imagining shutters closing over your third eye.*
- *Take time to tease out the issues and themes that are coming down the ancestral line to you or other members of the family. It may be a day or two before an 'ah ha' moment occurs.*
- *Place appropriate crystals on the photograph to heal those issues and themes.*
- *Leave the layout in place until dowsing shows you that the healing intervention is complete.*
- *Perform an appropriate healing layout on yourself to ensure that the themes do not carry forward into future generations.*

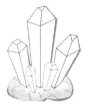

Healing the family tree

Systemic entanglements [are] said to occur when unresolved trauma has afflicted a family through an event such as murder, suicide, death of a mother in childbirth, early death of a parent or sibling, war, natural disaster, emigration, or abuse. The psychiatrist Iván Böszörményi-Nagy referred to this phenomenon as Invisible Loyalties.[17]

Quite apart from the effect of inherited ancestral memory, our earliest relationships are made within the family and may well reactivate our karmic expectations. They will certainly influence our adult relationships, social and familial. And they will definitely reflect the relationship style that has passed down the generations before us. Some families are loving and supportive, nurturing those in their midst. Others, sadly, are not but it is never too late to reverse the effect. Crystals generate an even more loving atmosphere within a loving family, or heal the results of lack of love in an indifferent or abusive one. Most emotional problems that families face have been passed down through the ancestral line, child learning from parent and passing it on, not knowing anything different – a situation which needs immense forgiveness and compassion. Using a simple visualisation and the assistance of a crystal, the whole family line can be reprogrammed to enjoy love and project it forward to future generations.

Ritual: Healing the Ancestral Line

If you have an actual family tree use it for this ritual, which reaches way back into the prehistory of the family, otherwise find a picture of an actual tree with deep root, visualise one or use the illustration on page 237. Dedicate your crystal to heal the whole family line.

You will need:

Ancestral healer crystal from the list
Family tree or the illustration on page 237
Most potent time: Full moon

Ritual: Ancestral healing

- *Holding your ancestral healer crystal, picture yourself leaning against a huge tree (or see yourself in your position on your family tree). The branches are present and future generations, the roots the ancestors.*
- *Place the healing stone at the bottom of the deepest taproot, or the start of the family tree. Tell yourself that this is the place of healing for the family as you stand your crystal here.*
- *Feel the crystal emanating forgiveness and loving compassion up through the roots, into the trunk and up*

into the branches, reprogramming negative family patterns as it goes.

- Roll that love out into branches and leaves that haven't developed yet for the benefit of future generations. Seed gifts for future generations into the branches.
- Bring that love and healing into your own heart.
- Leave the stone in place at the roots to continue the healing.
- You can extend this exercise by laying further crystals on the branches, trunk and roots of the tree as appropriate.

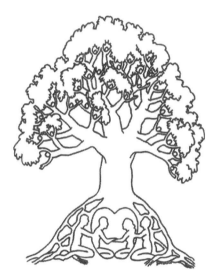

The family tree

Practical example:

14: Healing the family tree layout.
Ancestralite, Flint, Lakelandite, Rose Quartz,
Celtic Quartz and Eye of the Storm.

OR

OR: CAPTION Illustration 14: Healing the Tears of a
Nation (ritual for the dispossessed), Knowlton Henges,
summer 2016.

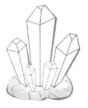

The Tree of Life

The sephirot, which are finite and measurable, are not, however, static objects, like fixed, solid rungs on the ladder of the progressive revelation of the divine attributes. They are, on the contrary, dynamic forces, ascending and descending, and extending themselves within the area of the Godhead. This dynamism is found both in their hidden existence, which is oriented upwards towards En-Sof, and also in their association with the lower world, as forces of creation and direction of the universe. They are in continuous motion, involved in innumerable processes of interweaving, interlinking, and union. Even their order changes as a result of their internal movement, and "their end is fastened into their beginning".

Tishby, commentary in *Wisdom of the Zohar*

The Kabbalistic Tree of Life is a symbolic representation of a multidimensional realm encompassing ten interconnected spheres, linked by 22 pathways. It is divided into four worlds:

- The supernal world beyond which is the ain, or nothing. 'The Source'.

- The creative world of archetypes and ideals.
- The formative world. The power of manifestation.
- Manifest creation, the material world.

The Tree is considered to be a map of the universe and the psyche, the order of the creation of the cosmos, and a path to spiritual illumination. But it is not necessary to go into these realms in depth in order to utilise the Tree for a past life or ancestral healing intervention as it takes you back to a primal, original and infinite energy state.

Ancestralite resonates particularly well with this layout, but you can use any of the healing stones that dowse as appropriate. Dowse for the order in which to lay the stones. You can either lay them over the body and the chakras – the crown, heart, sacral and base or base and earth star form the 'backbone' with the other spheres linking into other chakras. Alternatively, place over an ancestral tree or photograph.

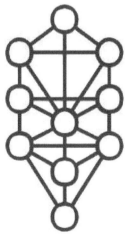

The Kabbalistic Tree of Life is an integral part of the Flower of Life, see the following page.

The Kabbalistic Tree of Life. Lay crystals in the order that intuitively feels appropriate for you and join up the grid with a crystal wand or the power of your mind.

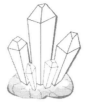

The Flower of Life

You can use the Flower of Life as a basis for personal or family healing, laying healing and detoxing crystals intuitively in whatever pattern feels right to you. It is called the Flower of Life because it, quite literally, encompasses the building blocks of life in one perfect form. The Flower of Life includes templates for the five Platonic Solids: primal patterns occurring within crystals – and life – everywhere. To the Greeks, these solids symbolised the elements of fire, earth, air, water, and spirit (universe or ether) respectively.

Although represented on the page in one dimension, the Flower of Life is actually multidimensional incorporating timelines and timeframes from past, present and future in addition to encompassing all the subtle bodies and the web woven by the ancestors. It can reach deep into the physical body, or the etheric bodies including the karmic and the ancestral, to entrain them back into harmony. So, the Flower of Life is useful as a background for layouts to radiate healing energy right through the ancestral line: past, present and future. The geometry of the Flower is such that it also incorporates many geometric grids such the Star of David and the complex Star of David, or the pentagram. All of which enhance the effect of the crystals on the ancestral line as they detox and pull in light. If you do not have a Flower of Life layout, use the one on the page opposite. Simply tune in and allow the crystals to do their work. Hold the intention that it will be for the highest good of all.

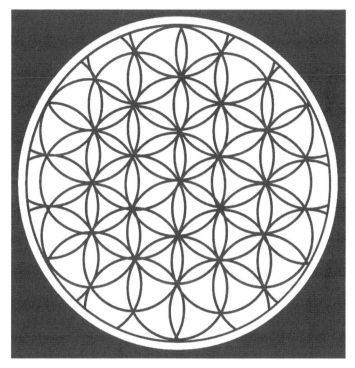

The Flower of Life

Practical example

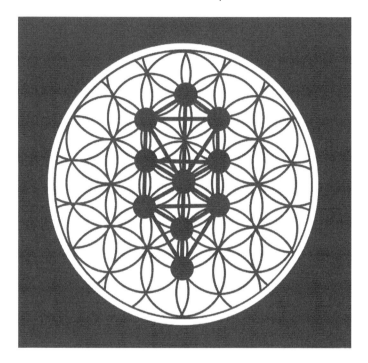

Intuitive Flower of Life laid out at an Ancestral Clearing
workshop with Cradle of Life, Rhodozite and Amethyst

Useful grids for the Flower of Life

Join up the points with a crystal wand or the power of your mind.

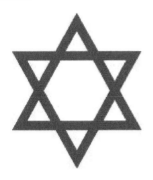

Star of David

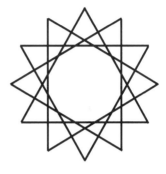

Complex Star of David

Pentagram

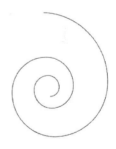

Spiral

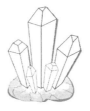

Re-weaving the web of family relationships

If you come from a broken or disrupted family line, re-weaving the web of family relationships is potent, but it is helpful for all families as it draws the members closer together in an unconditionally loving way. The power of the mind's eye to visualise is very potent in this ritual.

You will need:

A large dreamcatcher or spider's web (buy one or make your own)

Crystal beads

Most potent time: New moon

Ritual: Re-weaving the ancestral web

- *Using a dreamcatcher or spider's web, trace the outline with your eyes moving from the centre outwards. At the same time, imagine with your mind's eye that you are weaving the web that holds the family together with unconditional love. Whenever you find a piece of the web that is damaged or broken, run your finger along the dreamcatcher and imagine that you are mending the web. Attach a crystal on to the web you are working with wherever there is a break in the imagined one.*

- *When the whole web has been rewoven and repaired, place a Rose Quartz or Mangano Calcite in the centre of the actual web and picture it sending out the pink light of unconditional love and regard throughout the web on every level. Feel that love going back through the family and forward into generations to come.*
- *Decorate the dreamcatcher or web with appropriate crystal beads to bring healing and positive qualities to the family. Name each quality as you attach it.*
- *Hang it where you see it often.*

Alternatively: Place the crystals on the timeline web on page 185.

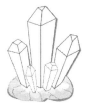

Transform negative family traits

Styles of parenting have a powerful effect on children and are, of course, passed down through families. Over-strictness is as damaging to a child as too much laxity. A child needs to learn how to live within but also how to set personal boundaries, how to tolerate frustration and take risks – all while feeling loved and supported by a parent. In that way, a child develops self-confidence and a feeling of being lovable that carries through into adult relationships.

Families carry emotional patterns such as repression – or explosions – of anger down through generations. Many have a list of 'forbidden feelings' that are not allowed expression: anger, lust, greed, sadness and such like. Others induce guilt or a sense of not being good enough. Some families have a repeating saga of early death or abandonment by a parent, of betrayal, secrecy or alcoholism or shame. The permutations are endless but are healed by sending forgiveness and compassion down the family line and sending love forward for the benefit of present and future generations (see overleaf).

Whilst closeness and intimacy are helpful in a family, too much of either may be intrusive and counterproductive. The child feels smothered. Equally damaging is the feeling that 'nobody cares'. Strombolite or Rose Quartz facilitates family healing as it fosters closeness and understanding without suffocation. Dedicate a large piece and place it in the centre of the family home.

Healing family myths

Families have their particular stories that play out time and time again through the generations. Superiority and inferiority often form the base of a family myth, as does betrayal or abandonment. If the family feels superior, no one else is good enough. If the family feels inferior, anyone who pays attention to a family member cannot be 'good'. Sacrifice is also a family myth: 'you must sacrifice yourself for the good of others' – this is closely allied to martyrdom. But families also have myths around love. 'Love hurts' is a scenario that gets passed from mother to daughter. 'Love has to be perfect' is often passed from mother to son – and the unspoken inference is that mother love is perfect and nothing else matches up. If your family carries such a myth, healing the ancestral line (see page 236) is a potent way to change it. Crystal EFT tapping (see page 104) can transform negative myths into positive affirmations of life.

Carrying tumbled stones assists family members to have positive beliefs about themselves and the family. Supportive tumbled stones, dedicated for the purpose, carried in the pocket or slipped under a pillow at night encourage positive attitudes.

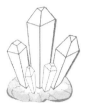

Releasing the family scapegoat

One person acting out a pattern or carrying the family burden saves the rest of the family from taking responsibility for their own behaviour and feelings. Family scapegoats tend to do all they can to placate their family and are forever trying to please and win approbation – or cut off all contact. They tend to act as victims or martyrs and are helped by the stones or gem essences for releasing those conditions (see page 321). But, when scapegoats take control of their own life, it causes enormous resistance from the family whose nice cosy illusion of 'I'm OK, it's not me that's the problem' is shattered.

Although it is an opportunity for the whole family to change, the scapegoat is often shunned when they begin to take control of their own life, pressurised to 'return to normal', or someone else in the family takes on the role. Ideally all the family would be involved in healing a scapegoating pattern but may refuse due to resistance to change. However, it is possible to 'reprogram' the family from afar by distance healing with a crystal. Some people might feel that this interferes in the family free will. But, did anyone ask the scapegoat if they wanted that role? The reply is usually that it was thrust upon them and may well be a karmic carry-over. Assisting the scapegoat facilitates a change they or the family may not be capable of bringing about for themselves and gives the whole family an opportunity to move on.

You will need:

Family photograph
Rose Quartz or Selenite
Scapolite or other scapegoating crystal
Most potent time: Full moon

Ritual: Healing the family scapegoat

- *Place a photograph of the whole family in a place where it will not be disturbed and preferably where the light from the full moon will fall on it. Surround it with Rose Quartz or Celtic Quartz (white for the matrilineal line, Golden for the patriarchal) crystals.*
- *Over the family scapegoat, place a scapegoat healer stone such as Scapolite.*
- *Now visualise pink light surrounding that person, or yourself. If you are the scapegoat, say out loud: "I am not responsible for the problems and feelings of my family. The family situation is not my creation. I am responsible only for myself." If you are not the scapegoat, use: "We/you are not responsible."*
- *Repeat night and morning for a week.*

- *If jealousy or other toxic emotions are involved, drop appropriate gem essences on to the crystal (see pages 123–127).*

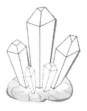

Generational curses

In 16th century Turkey it was believed that if you disturbed a djinn at night you would be left 'crippled until doomsday'. And, what's more, the curse would be so strong that it would last for seven generations. Let's look at that a moment. A generation is deemed to be between 20–25 years. That covers a span of between 140 and 175 years. Quite long enough to be firmly imprinted in the 'junk DNA' especially if it became a family saga: "Your seven times great-grandmother went out to the privy in the night and disturbed a djinn. Her leg and arm withered and eventually she died. That happened to Great-aunt Ayla too. Be careful or it could happen to you." Similar superstitions are to be found around the world.

The ancient concept of generational curses is an ingrained component of religion and may in itself create a susceptibility or a thought form that passes through a family. In the Hebrew bible such curses occur several times with "a jealous God, punishing the children for the sin of the fathers to the third and fourth generation". This is based on the idea that family lifestyles are likely to pass down through the generations so the same 'sins' will be repeated with future generations compounding those of the ancestors. The curse will be firmly imprinted by the time of the fourth or fifth generation (Exodus 20:5, 34:7; Numbers 14:18; Deuteronomy 5:9). Some of the curses are petty comprehensive and it's hardly surprising that Jews can be found scattered to the four corners of the Earth given what their ancestors were led to expect. But all the Abrahamic faiths have this concept built into their foundations:

But it shall come to pass, if thou wilt not hearken unto the voice of the LORD thy God, to observe to do all his commandments and his statutes which I command thee this day; that all these curses shall come upon thee, and overtake thee: [16]Cursed shalt thou be in the city, and cursed shalt thou be in the field. [17]… thy basket and thy store. [18]… the fruit of thy body, and the fruit of thy land, the increase of thy kine, and the flocks of thy sheep. [19]… thou be when thou comest in, and cursed shalt thou be when thou goest out. [20]The LORD shall send upon thee cursing, vexation, and rebuke, in all that thou settest thine hand unto for to do, until thou be destroyed, and until thou perish quickly; because of the wickedness of thy doings, whereby thou hast forsaken me. [21]… make the pestilence cleave unto thee, until he have consumed thee from off the land, whither thou goest to possess it. [22]… smite thee with a consumption, and with a fever, and with an inflammation, and with an extreme burning, and with the sword, and with blasting, and with

mildew; and they shall pursue thee until thou perish. [23]...
[24]*... make the rain of thy land powder and dust: from heaven shall it come down upon thee, until thou be destroyed.* [25]*...* [27]*... smite thee with the botch of Egypt, and with the emerods, and with the scab, and with the itch, whereof thou canst not be healed.* [28]*... with madness, and blindness, and astonishment of heart...*

And so on for another 60 verses until:

[66]*And thy life shall hang in doubt before thee; and thou shalt fear day and night, and shalt have none assurance of thy life:* [67]*...* [68]*... and there ye shall be sold unto your enemies for bondmen and bondwomen, and no man shall buy you.*

Deuteronomy 28:15–68, King James Authorised Version (www.kingjamesbibleonline.org)

Time for a change wouldn't you say? It is in this way that family scapegoats and the sense of a 'cursed family line' are built into ancestral memory and 'junk DNA'. It makes no difference if two, two hundred or two thousand years have passed. The effect is embedded and needs to be rooted out.

The Uncursing Ritual

This ritual is excellent for removing past life curses that hold a soul part in thrall but it also clears ancestral curses and attachments, thought forms and spirits. You can do it for yourself or on another person.

- *Place four Tourmalinated Quartz or Purpurite crystals at each corner of a rectangle large enough to lie down in (using a cloth to outline the space is helpful). Join the crystals up with a wand to create a sacred space into which you can step or place the person with whom you are working. The ritual is best conducted lying down.*
- *Place a fifth Tourmalinated Quartz or Purpurite crystal just below the breastbone above the solar plexus. Hold a Nuummite crystal in your right hand (a wand or wedge shape is ideal) and a Novaculite or Flint shard in your left hand.*
- *Beginning at the crown chakra, place both hands above the head and 'comb' across the chakra about a hand's breadth above the body with each of the crystals in turn starting with the Novaculite (be careful as this flinty crystal can be very sharp). As you work on the chakra, ask that you or the person you are working on and all the ancestral line be released from all and any curses/thought forms that have been put at any time in the past.*
- *Moving your hands in a figure of eight formation that crosses and then moves apart again at each chakra, move down the body cleansing and clearing each chakra in turn.*
- *When you reach the base chakra, work back up the chakras again with the same sweeping figure of eight movement until you reach the crown. Continue until*

the chakras feel clear.

- *Now close your eyes and ask that the person who placed the curse will make him or herself known to you. You may see a clear picture or get a prickling sensation on one side of your head or a pain somewhere in your body – in which case move the Tourmalinated Quartz over the spot either on your own body or that of your patient to absorb the pain. Talk to this person, discuss why the curse was placed, how it can be removed and what reparation, if any, is required on either side. Offer and accept forgiveness. Then ask that the curse be lifted from the recipient and all the generations to come and those who have gone before, everyone who has been affected. Feel the effect of the crystals radiating back through time and forward into the future freed from the effects of the curse and bringing beneficial experiences and joyful learning to everyone involved.*

- *Work through each charka in turn with the Novaculite and Nuummite again, healing and sealing each one with light.*

- *Find a place where you can set out the grid and leave it to continue its work.*

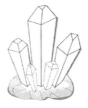

Ancestral Case History: Powerful happenings in the night

I am including this case history because it brings together so many facets: family history, toxic emotions, thought forms, personal experience and more. Of necessity the writer has to remain anonymous but it is someone I have known for a number of years. Several different modes of healing intervention were involved and I was not the only person working on the complex case. Each approach added, or subtracted, another layer, bringing another level of understanding and release to the overall whole. As I didn't take notes of the crystals I used, I have to rely on what was noted by the participant at the time. But my abiding memory is of the Rose Quartz skull and the unconditional love with which it enfolded every player throughout the process as I communicated with the suspended soul and the family line, and supported the lineage breaker in his task.

My father died in 2012. When clearing out his belongings, my sister came across a framed photograph of his elder brother in military dress uniform. She brought the photograph to me saying she was going to throw it out. I knew immediately that that was the wrong thing to do and said that it would be like throwing a person away. My uncle had died in 1941 at the age of 21 and there was no one else to remember him. The death of my uncle and a number of otherwise untimely deaths in the family hung around my childhood – not spoken about much, but there. Accordingly, I stood the picture in my kitchen. She also gave me my father's watches, one of which belonged to my uncle. It still worked although its timing was erratic. I kept it next to my bed. It stopped at one minute past 5 and stayed at that time. The photograph and the watch moved with me in 2014. I did not pay any particular attention to either of them. I think that as they both related to my uncle they were useful in connecting me to him and in bringing what follows in this story to the surface.

I will have to refer in this story to the sex urge if it is to make any sense. It is important to relate that, having been brought up in a very free and easy environment, I have never at any stage had any anxiety about or around sex or the perfor-mance of same – although it has been a powerful force with me being a Leo sun sign with Scorpio rising. I am gay. My family made very little fuss over that but, when realising at the age of 13 or so that I was gay, I knew immediately that I would have to spend a life effectively in hiding and learning to fly under the radar. Shame and self-hatred over this issue started at that time. However, the realisation of the power of the sex instinct gave a sense of immediate compensation and I came to see the two elements as being part of the same thing.

In 2015, I went on a course of Psychic Development. The essence of the course was how to raise one's vibration to work clairvoyantly at the level of the brow chakra. By the fourth and final session, each of the group had to do a clairvoyant reading in front of the class and the tutor. I had noticed between the third and fourth sessions that I had started to become notably anxious around the subject of sex. A casual but intense encounter had laid me really low and appeared to open me up. When my turn came, I was quite nervous and specifically told myself to "open my third eye". The tutor asked, "What can you see?" I had a quick glimpse of my uncle – visible by his uniform – walking down a street in the sunshine. I was looking at him from the rear and the image was extremely thin. I told the tutor I could see a member of my family but she told me that I was supposed to be finding someone relevant to the other people in the room. So the image of my uncle disappeared and was replaced by a very black face in a pork pie hat – not a black man but the whole image being black – with huge eye sockets like a skull. I didn't recognise him and no one in the room picked up my description. The two images were markedly different – one a figure like a needle taking up very little space and the other completely filling my vision.

Immediately after the class, I knew that something had happened to my sexual energy. It was as though it had disappeared – along with all physical functioning. It was as though I had been hit hard in the genitalia with a soft mallet. Judy subsequently told me that this was a transferred memory of a blow my uncle had received during the injuries that led to his death, which is referred to later. The next day after I sat for an hour in a meeting, I realised I had lost all sensation in that area. It was as though all blood circulation had gone and I had to spend the day trying to revive any feeling at all. I was relieved to get some sensation back but everything else had completely disappeared. Like a sort of trauma.

So, suddenly, from having been perfectly well, I realised I was in a mess. As one consultant said, I had blown all my fuses. I felt I would never regain my sexual health. The two images I saw did not seem to have any particular relevance at the time – only the physiological effect. One thing I realised later is that I was not grounded at all. I had failed in the method I was using and was completely unconnected. That was a lesson for me.

Anxiety took me over in a big way. I rushed into action with all sorts of healing and therapy – basically anything that might help. The first thing I did, following a curious series of circumstances (which I can now see was part of the journey), was to contact a friend of mine, David. I had known him for a number of years and knew he did energy work. He told me I should look at my sexual history and how I had used sex; have a period of abstinence and that it was imperative that I did work releasing old contracts/templates/patterns – anything that I held that was no longer necessary and useful – or indeed truthful. I would have to change as the old was no longer working. He said this was something that was being experienced by many people at the present time and that I was at least on the button with it coming to my attention. He started that process for me and I found I could do it quite easily on my own. I continued it over several sessions. I felt the old contracts releasing like the pinging of elastic bands held at tension inside me.

Within two weeks of the class, I also had an extraordinary dream which involved a series of images of death and which I wrote down at the time as "powerful happenings in the night": looking up a rope from which I was being hanged; screaming and terror; the word garrotting; lots of restrictions around the neck; a dead face lying on a velvet pillow; Charles the First; Egypt; finding myself locked alone in a room tied to a chair and shouting if anyone was there; going to a house and looking for an old entrance (now removed) which somehow led to all this. A strong sense of things being uncovered. I woke up and felt huge amounts of warm heat rolling through me. It took a long time and I just lay there in the heat accepting it. I was very surprised indeed to experience this phenomenon as I have not spent a great deal of time considering healing. But I realised I had been receiving it in a big way. As regards the series of death images, were these my deaths or perhaps a mix of mine and others of my ancestors or indeed those of other people? I don't know. It would make sense that they are somehow connected to me but David (ever practical) told me not to spend time on the detail. We have all had many deaths, he said.

Two weeks later, I had another strange experience in the night. When I tried to go to sleep, I started to feel quite depressed and a huge number of images started to fill my vision. It was constant for some hours but I couldn't really see what any of it was. It seemed to be black and white and was like a mass of interference or a code (not to be understood for itself) and millions of bits of images all mixed up and jumbled and moving really quickly. There was I think an element of sound to it as well. I managed to get some sleep and when I woke at 6am, it had stopped and my mind was noticeably quiet. I was hugely relieved. It became clear over the next few days that this was not just the content of one life but of many lives and it was like a computer emptying itself. I realised that I had been undergoing a huge clearance of information held by me – and maybe of others.

Throughout this, I charted my state of mind through the prism of my sexual functioning and my levels of anxiety. I found myself very much in the world of comparing myself with others and feeling infinitely inferior and worn out. I mourned my life before I had the experience as though I could never regain it. David asked me: "Are you up for this? Can you just surrender to going with it? That is the best thing if you can find the courage." By a series of circumstances, I became aware that I had been knocked out of my body and had blown open my third eye. Accordingly, the etheric body had to be realigned with the physical and the third eye issue dealt with. After that, I started to feel better though still anxious. I thought the crisis had passed.

However, by February 2016, I realised I was getting worse again. It was as though something was leeching all my sexual energy. My anxiety was at an all-time high. Someone told me I had an attachment and I went to have it removed. However, I felt worse than ever. Having had a sort of recovery, I didn't know what to do. Someone suggested that I contact Judy, who I had known for many years. I had already confided in her some of my experiences during this episode and she had confirmed that I had indeed been knocked out of my body. Accordingly, I told her that I seemed to have gone back to where I was and she wrote: "Clearly something more is going on. Can you think back to anyone in your ancestral line who may have been either sex addicted or 'sex starved'? I keep getting a strong sense of that being passed down the transgenerational line and that someone is feeding on your sexual energy." She told me that the person she was getting wouldn't have talked about it and I should look at my family history and make an intuitive leap. I coursed around through my family history. The experiences I had had in the class came immediately to mind but I tried to hide from them – they felt too sensitive. However, Judy said that was a good place to start and it rapidly became clear that that was what I should concentrate on.

Accordingly, I set up a session with Judy for the beginning of March. In the days leading up to the event, around the photograph and the watch, I gathered a number of crystals that I had lying around the house – from memory, a Quartz crystal obelisk with rainbows, several pieces of Carnelian Agate, pieces of Obsidian and Rhodonite, some Preseli Bluestone, Citrine and a Lapis Lazuli skull. Plus two crystals, Ancestralite and Celtic Golden Healer, that Judy had said were perfect for releasing – I had attended an ancestral clearing workshop with her as a preliminary to the individual session. I said to the crystals: I don't know what any of you do but I need you to help me and my uncle with this event. It was clear that they clustered around the photograph and watch and immediately started to do this. I took them to the sitting.

We laid them on the table. Judy had brought with her a Rose

Quartz skull but for the operation itself used a large piece of Malachite. I had told her that my uncle had been found in a communal shower with very strange injuries and that shortly afterwards he had died. I had heard rumblings in my family that the death was not straightforward but the details were scarce as it had happened during wartime and, even though we found a mound of correspondence about it in my father's belongings, the exact cause remained elusive. Nothing really is known and there is no way to find out. However, Judy and I have been able to intuit that rather than it involving matters of a purely sexual nature, more it involved the crossing of gender divides as we commonly understand them. Beyond that we cannot establish.

Indeed, it has become clear to me that the specifics are not particularly relevant anyway, except for the underlying element of shame. What did become apparent from the sitting was that my uncle had been 'in suspension' since the event of his death. I thought originally that he was stuck but Judy said no, just suspended – time, of course, not having the same relevance as it does to us. It is a curious fact, looking back and entirely with the benefit of hindsight, that a photograph of him that hung in my Grandma's house had him looking very handsome – but somehow as though stuck in glass. I can well believe that, to my family, if they had any realisation of these circumstances, they (like many others at the time) would be most unlikely to have been able to confront it and, if known, would probably have hidden from it.

Judy first had to release my uncle but rather clandestinely because it was important that she did not disturb the second character that I had encountered, who otherwise might have tried to hide. It seems he was a thought form who had jumped in when I had banged myself completely open doing the mediumship. Once my uncle was freed, Judy was able to disperse the thought form so that we could turn our attention to my uncle.

My uncle had died before he had been able to have any sexual experiences of his own and he, and the thought form, had been vicariously locked into my sexual energy, draining it. I was rather spooked by this until Judy said she had spoken to my uncle about it and he said, "Well he did agree to it." Or at least, so far as he himself was concerned. The thought form was a hitchhiker attracted by the intense energy of the sexual encounter I had had during my psychic training. That makes complete sense and I thought it was quite funny. It became the relatively routine matter of an agreement between two people/souls and I felt reassured by it. Nobody had taken any advantage of anybody. It seems obvious to me now that having personally experienced the difficulties of a relatively non routine sexuality myself, but living in an era in which it has become very easy in the main to deal with it, I am a suitable person to deal with the issue of shame – especially of the sort it seems he and the family may have experienced.

After the session, we noticed that the Malachite had a crack running through it which neither of us had noticed before. It had clearly opened up with the force of what Judy had to do, creating a portal. I also noted a few days later that the watch had moved on to just before 5.15. I took home with me the Rose Quartz skull that Judy had also used to assist my uncle to heal and to send reassurance and forgiveness down the ancestral line.

At Judy's suggestion, as we did not have time for further work, I went immediately to another consultant who told me that in his opinion I had been around my uncle in a number of other lives. Something Judy later confirmed. It makes sense to me that, in these circumstances, I would certainly recognise unconsciously when presented with the photograph that it should not be thrown away. I realised also as time went by that, as I was not born until 15 years after he had died, most probably I had come to know of his condition and had made a life contract somehow to release him from it prior to my current incarnation. Of course, consciously, I would not know this. It has taken some time for the circumstances to be right for me to do it. It seems strange that it happened through the prism of sex, but it also makes sense. As Judy said, "They had to draw your attention to it somehow."

But there is another dimension to this. I come from a family who, even though some members on both sides have had a number of psychic experiences, have in the main not wanted to engage with it – even though I have to a marked degree. However, Judy told me quite recently that in the past some of my ancestors have used their psychic skills – but not for the best motives. It makes sense then that this has set up a resistance and shame around the subject in my family, as with the sexual element. It became clear that what I was being called on to do was to face up to the shame element in my ancestors and possibly effect a release for them from it. I see shame as being a general concept. I realise I have to do it on a personal level and *need to stop buying into this generalised shame that I have experienced, and also do it for them.*

Judy has recently explained to me the concept of the lineage breaker. It had seemed strange to me that, coming as I do from the same family as my siblings and other family members, I have not shown the same distrust of the psychic world as they have – indeed completely the opposite.

So now I find myself at the crossroads between the past and future of my line with the responsibility of looking after both those who have gone before and those still to come. I was initially hesitant to write this story – especially as it is to find its way into a book – but after some initial resistance from my ancestors, they have come to acknowledge that we need to complete this release. Otherwise, we will remain locked in by the concept of shame. If we don't face up to it, the opportunity will be missed and it may not come again for a long time. I may indeed be the lineage breaker. My experience is that we have to get away from sticking with ideas and thoughts that are outdated to our generation and are no longer really of benefit to anyone. As I wrote, I hoped I was not making a mistake and asked the Rose Quartz skull to assist me. As the day has gone on, I have felt more and more that not to do this would be a greater error. I offer it in the hope that it will assist other people.

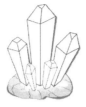

Ancestral house clearing

All but the newest of houses have an ancestral history – and even then the land on which a new dwelling is built may well have an ancestral saga attached. All the owners and occupiers who have lived there throughout the years will have left their energetic mark: their joys and sorrows, hopes and expectations, fear and fantasies. Tie cutting may be needed to free up the energies. Houses can be 'happy' or 'sad' places. Especially when larger spaces have been carved up into smaller units or the building has undergone a change of use. Sometimes this energetic residue chimes with our own, which is why a house can reach out and grab you. Make you feel you've 'come home'. Or, a building may repel you because it mirrors your own or your ancestors' less than beneficial past experience. The house may have much to teach you.

Houses can also hold on to the horrors of the past. In the UK, as with other places, many old asylums, prisons and former poorhouses, religious or commercial buildings have been converted into flats. Occupants often report disturbances that can be traced back to the despair, beliefs or psychosis of former inmates. In some cases, the previous occupants are still there and need help to move on (see page 214). In other cases the desperation has been imprinted into the walls and floors, seeping into the very foundations and land on which a building stands. An imprint that may not be dissolved if a building is torn down or decays. Traumatic events such as battles, family quarrels, or turning the occupants off the land may also have left their mark. The actions of thoughtless and unaware property developers may lead to problems further down the line in the present day. One former church, for instance, had had the occupants of the graves disinterred and the bones thrown into the crypt, which was then walled up. The restless souls soon made themselves known when a sensitive owner moved in.

Healing ancestral patterns in houses

One of the quickest ways of healing the ancestral memory of a building is by using crystal layouts combined with essences such as Petaltone Z14 or Astral Clear (see Resources). If you do not have enough crystals of any one type, crystals can be mixed, or you can make a crystal essence and use that.

You will need:

Sufficient cleansed Ancestralite or other ancestral clearing stones for each corner of every room in the building. Crystal types can be mixed as long as the outermost four corners have Ancestralite placements.

Keep the overall crystal placements harmonious and symmetrical.
A large Selenite sphere
Petaltone Z14 or Astral Clear

- *Ground yourself thoroughly with a grounding root. (See page 19.)*
- *Programme the crystals with the intention that they will clear and heal the ancestral history of the building and release any trapped souls to the light.*
- *Place large Ancestralite stones in the four outermost corners of the building.*
- *Place appropriate crystals in each corner of every room, keeping an overall pattern and symmetry to the placements depending in the shape of the building.*
- *Place a large Selenite sphere as close as possible to the centre of the building.*
- *Put a few drops of Petaltone Z14, Astral Clear or other ancestral clearing essence on each of the Ancestralites in the outer corners and on the central Selenite sphere.*
- *Send unconditional love and forgiveness right through the building as you visualise all the crystals joining up in a multidimensional grid that sends clearing and healing light from top to bottom and side to side and then down into the land beneath.*
- *If issues or emotions surface, add appropriate crystals to the grid.*
- *Leave the crystals in place for as long as feels appropriate. Spray with crystal cleanser from time to time*

and then thoroughly cleanse them when dismantling the grid.

Alternatively, the quick method:

- *Lay a large five pointed star grid using ancestral clearing crystals in the centre of the space with a Selenite sphere in the centre.*
- *Place Rose Quartz between the ancestral stones and the Selenite at the crossing point of the lines.*
- *Add appropriate crystal essences to each stone.*
- *Visualise the crystals joining up in a multidimensional grid that sends clearing and healing light from top to bottom and side to side of the space and then down into the land beneath.*
- *Ask that any lost souls be taken to the light.*
- *Leave the crystals in place for as long as feels appropriate.*

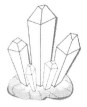

Honouring the ancestors

In traditional societies, ancestors are an honoured part of the family. Ancient peoples kept bones under the floor, created home altars, or regularly visited tombs making offerings so that the spirits of the ancestors blessed them. In modern families people often unknowingly make an equivalent 'family altar' with displays of photographs or inherited objects (which may need to be cleansed, see page 218). An altar can be used to honour and bless the ancestors and to bring their blessings into your everyday life. Spirit Quartz is an ancestor-orientated stone as is Ancestralite.

You will need:

Family photographs
Large photograph frame
Spirit and Rose Quartz or Ancestralite
Tea light or candle in holder
Most potent time: Full moon

Ritual: Honouring the ancestors

- *Gather together a selection of family photographs that*

span the generations and create a collage radiating out with you or your immediate family in the centre. As you do so, thank each person for being part of your ancestral line and ask for their blessing.

- *Frame the collage and set it up in the ancestral portion of your home (the middle of the left-hand wall of the house).*
- *Light the candle and place it in front of the collage.*
- *Hold the Spirit Quartz or Ancestralite and dedicate it to honouring your ancestors. Touch each ancestor with the crystal and bless them. Place the crystal in front of the collage.*
- *If you feel that more love is needed, place Rose Quartz next to the Spirit Quartz.*
- *As you blow the candle out, send love, blessings and honour out through future generations.*

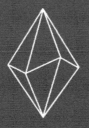

Part V
A–Z Directory

Crystals for karmic healing,
soul reintegration
and ancestral clearing

– A –

Abandonment, overcome feelings of: Cassiterite, Chalcanthite, Golden Healer, Quantum Quattro, Rhodochrosite, Rhodozaz, Rhodozite, Rose Quartz, Tugtupite. *Chakra:* base, three-chambered heart

Abuse: Apricot Quartz, Aventurine, Azeztulite with Morganite, Eilat Stone, Golden Healer, Honey Opal, Lazurine, Lemurian Jade, Morganite with Azeztulite, Pink Crackle Quartz, Proustite, Red Quartz, Rhodolite Garnet, Rhodonite, Septarian, Shiva Lingam, Shiva Shell, Smoky Amethyst, Smoky Citrine, Xenotine. *Chakra:* base, sacral, three-chambered heart

> **break away from:** Cradle of Life (Humankind), Freedom Stone, Rhodolite Garnet, Rhodonite, Xenotine. *Chakra:* sacral and solar plexus

> **clear emotional:** Apricot Quartz, Aventurine, Azeztulite with Morganite, Cradle of Life (Humankind), Honey Opal, Lazurine, Mount Shasta Opal, Rose Quartz, Rosophia, Smoky Rose Quartz, Tugtupite, Xenotine. *Chakra:* sacral, heart

> **sexual, heal:** Apricot Quartz, Eilat Stone, Golden Healer, Proustite, Rhodolite Garnet, Rhodonite, Shiva Lingam. *Chakra:* base, sacral

Acceptance of physical body: Bloodstone, Celestobarite, Cradle of Life (Humankind), Empowerite, Golden Healer, Keyiapo, Llanite (Llanoite), Moldavite, Quantum Quattro, Que Sera, Rhodolite Garnet, Riebekite with Sugilite and Bustamite, Schalenblende, Thompsonite, and see Incarnation page 332. *Chakra:* earth star, base, dantien, crown

Accepting oneself: see Self-acceptance page 366

Addiction: Amethyst, Amethyst Elestial Quartz, Aventurine, Azurite, Banded Agate, Black Tourmaline, Blue Fluorite, Blue Topaz, Botswana Agate, Brandenberg Amethyst, Carnelian, Celestite, Citrine, Crackled Fire Agate, Danburite, Fenster Quartz, Golden Selenite, Green Tourmaline, Hematite, Iolite, Kiwi Stone, Labradorite, Lazulite, Lepidolite, Malachite, Peridot, Quartz, Selenite, Smoky Amethyst, Smoky Quartz, Tantalite, Vera Cruz Amethyst. *Chakra:* base, sacral, dantien. Take as alcohol-free essence or carry at all times, or hold crystals with your hands in your groin creases.

   alcohol: Amazez, Amethyst, Auralite 23, Celestite (in right hand) and Celestite (in left)

   caffeine: Green Tourmaline, Malachite, Peridot, Quartz. *Chakra:* solar plexus

   chocolate: Amethyst, Citrine, Jasper

   cocaine: Angel's Wing Calcite, Aventurine (in right hand) and Selenite (in left hand), Azeztulite

   heroin: Aventurine (in left hand) and Selenite (in right hand), Lepidolite, Peridot

   marijuana: Anandalite, Azurite (in left hand) and Carnelian (in right hand), Carnelian

   sexual: Anandalite, Blue Topaz, Garnet, Kundalini Quartz, Poppy Jasper, Rhodonite, Serpentine

   sugar: Clear Quartz (in right hand) and Rose Quartz (in left hand), Drusy Quartz, Rhodochrosite, Spirit

Quartz

tobacco: Blue Fluorite (in left hand) and Smoky Quartz (in right hand), Botswana Agate

Note: Keep crystals in pocket when not in hands. Hand connections extracted from Donna Cunningham's Spiritual Dimensions of Healing Addictions*, see Resources.*

understand causes of: Auralite 23, Carnelian, Chrysotile, Crystal Cap Amethyst, Dumortierite, Fenster Quartz, Garnet, Iolite, Kornerupine, Malachite, Red Amethyst, Rose Quartz, Smoky Amethyst, Vera Cruz Amethyst. *Chakra:* past life, base, causal vortex

Aggression, ameliorate: Blizzard Stone, Fluorapatite, Pyrite in Magnesite, Rose Quartz, Sardonyx. *Chakra:* base, dantien

Akashic Record, read: Afghanite, Amphibole, Ancestralite, Andescine Labradorite, Blue Aventurine, Blue Euclase, Brandenberg Amethyst, Brookite, Cathedral Quartz, Celestial Quartz, Celestobarite, Chinese Writing Quartz, Chrysotile, Cradle of Life (Humankind), Datolite, Dumortierite, Eilat Stone, Heulandite, K2, Keyiapo, Lemurian Aquitane Calcite, Merkabite Calcite, Merlinite, Optical Calcite, Phosphosiderite, Prehnite, Prophecy Stone, Serpentine in Obsidian, Sichuan Quartz, Tanzanite, Tibetan Black Spot Quartz, Tremolite, Trigonic Quartz. *Chakra:* past life, third eye, crown, causal vortex

Alcoholism: Amethyst, Amethyst Elestial Quartz,

Auralite 23, Vera Cruz Amethyst, and see Addiction above. *Chakra:* base, sacral, past life

Alien or reptilian entities, release: Chlorite Quartz, Feather Pyrite, Jasper Knife, Rainbow Mayanite, Snakeskin Agate, Stibnite followed by Anandalite, Selenite, or Mica to seal the aura. Place over site of attachment.

Alienation, overcome: Amphibole Quartz, Bustamite with Sugilite, Cassiterite, Celtic Quartz, Champagne Aura Quartz, Cradle of Life (Humankind), Gaia Stone, Rhodochrosite, Rhodolite Garnet, Rose Quartz. *Chakra:* earth star, solar plexus, soma

Align self with spiritual energy: Anandalite, Andean Blue Opal, Annabergite, Celadonite, Ethiopian Opal, Lemurian Seed, Prophecy Stone, Ruby Lavender Quartz, Sillimanite. *Chakra:* crown, soul star, stellar gateway

Align soul with physical body: Ajo Blue Calcite, Anandalite, Cradle of Life (Humankind), Empowerite, Larvikite, Schalenblende, Scheelite, Scolecite, Sichuan Quartz, Sillimanite, Thompsonite. Hold over head or solar plexus.

Alta major chakra: Afghanite, Anandalite, Andara Glass, Angelinite, Angel's Wing Calcite, Apatite, Auralite 23, Aurichalcite, Azeztulite, Black Moonstone, Blue Kyanite, Blue Moonstone, Brandenberg Amethyst, Budd Stone (African Jade), Cradle of Life (Humankind), Crystal Cap Amethyst, Diaspore (Zultanite), Emerald, Ethiopian Opal, Eye of the Storm (Judy's Jasper), Fire and Ice Quartz, Flint, Fluorapatite, Garnet in Pyroxene, Golden

Healer, Golden Herkimer Diamond, Graphic Smoky Quartz, Green Ridge Quartz, Herkimer Diamond, Holly Agate, Hungarian Quartz, Petalite, Phenacite, Preseli Bluestone, Rainbow Covellite, Rainbow Mayanite, Red Agate, Red Amethyst, Rosophia. Place on base of skull.

balance and align: Anandalite, Blue Kyanite, Brandenberg Amethyst, Crystal Cap Amethyst, Green Ridge Quartz, Preseli Bluestone on soma chakra *and* Angel's Wing Calcite, Blue Kyanite, Flint or Herkimer Diamond on base of skull

spin too rapid/stuck open: Auralite 23, Black Moonstone, Blue Kyanite, Budd Stone (African Jade) Calcite, Eye of the Storm, Flint, Golden Healer, Graphic Smoky Quartz, Serpentine. Place at base of skull.

spin too sluggish/stuck closed: Blue Moonstone, Diaspore, Ethiopian Opal, Herkimer Diamond, Quartz, Red Agate, Serpentine, Triplite

Ancestral attachment/myths/stories carried in the genes: Anandalite, Ancestralite, Brandenberg Amethyst, Celtic Quartz, Cradle of Life (Humankind), Datolite, Fairy Quartz, Freedom Stone, Lakelandite, Lemurian Seed, Picture Jasper, Preseli Bluestone, Rainforest Jasper, Spirit Quartz, Smoky Elestial. *Chakra:* soma, causal vortex, solar plexus

Ancestral healer crystals: Ammolite, Ammonite, Anandalite, Ancestral healer (large crystal with a distinctive flat pathway running up the crystal from bottom to top), Ancestralite, Brandenberg, Celtic

Chevron Quartz, Chrysotile, Cradle of Life (Humankind), Dumortierite, Elestial Quartz, Fairy Quartz, Freedom Stone, Kambaba Jasper, Lakelandite, Mother and child formation (a large crystal to which is attached a smaller crystal or crystals that appears to be enfolded), Petrified Wood, Preseli Bluestone, Smithsonite, Smoky Elestial, Spirit Quartz, Stromatolite, Territula Agate, Wind Fossil Agate. *Chakra:* past life, causal vortex

Ancestral issues: Ancestralite, Celtic Quartz, Cradle of Life (Humankind), Golden Healer, Lakelandite, Porphyrite (Chinese Letter Stone). *Chakra:* past life, causal vortex, alta major

Ancestral line, healing: Amber, Ancestralite, Brandenberg Amethyst, Candle Quartz, Chlorite Quartz, Cradle of Life (Humankind), Crinoidal Limestone, Datolite, Fairy Quartz, Golden Healer, Ilmenite, Kambaba Jasper, Lemurian Aquitane Calcite, Mohawkite, Petrified Wood, Prasiolite, Rainforest Jasper, Shaman Quartz, Smoky Elestial Quartz, Spirit Quartz, Stromatolite. *Chakra:* past life, base, causal vortex

Ancestral patterns: Ancestralite, Anthrophyllite, Arfvedsonite, Candle Quartz, Celadonite, Celtic Quartz, Cradle of Life (Humankind), Crinoidal Limestone, Eclipse Stone, Garnet in Quartz, Glendonite, Golden Healer, Green Ridge Quartz, Holly Agate, Lakelandite, Mohawkite, Picture Jasper, Porphyrite (Chinese Letter Stone), Prasiolite, Rainbow Covellite, Rainbow Mayanite, Scheelite, Shaman Quartz with Chlorite, Starseed Quartz,

Wind Fossil Agate. *Chakra:* past life, causal vortex, alta major

Anger, ameliorate: Cinnabar in Jasper, Ethiopian Opal, Garnet, Nzuri Moyo. *Chakra:* base, dantien

Anger at God: Eudialyte, Rhodolite Garnet

Angst: Hemimorphite, Rhodonite, Rose Quartz

Anorexia from past life causes: Ancestralite, Azotic Topaz, Cradle of Life (Humankind), Lakelandite, Mystic Topaz, Orange Kyanite, Picasso Jasper, Tugtupite. *Chakra:* earth star, base, heart

Anxiety: Amethyst, Danburite, Galaxyite, Khutnohorite, Kunzite, Kyanite, Lemurian Aquitane Calcite, Lemurian Gold Opal, Lithium Quartz, Nzuri Moyo, Oceanite, Owyhee Blue Opal, Pinolith, Pyrite in Magnesite, Riebekite with Sugilite and Bustamite, Rose Quartz, Scolecite, Strawberry Quartz, Tanzanite, Thunder Egg, Tremolite, Tugtupite. *Chakra:* earth star, base

Apathy: Brookite, Bushman Red Cascade, Chinese Red Quartz, Macedonian Opal, Poppy Jasper, Zebra Stone. *Chakra:* base, sacral, dantien

Arrogance: Covellite, Diopside, Rhodolite Garnet. *Chakra:* base and soma

Arthritis: Ancestralite, Aztee, Blue Euclase, Brochantite, Calcite Fairy Stone, Chalcanthite, Chalcopyrite, Chinese Red Quartz, Chrysocolla, Dianite, Golden Healer, Malachite, Native Copper, Nzuri Moyo, Paraiba Tourmaline, Plancheite, Prophecy Stone, Rhodozite, Shungite, Turquoise, Wind Fossil Agate. Hold or wear constantly.

Assimilate change: Actinolite, Basalt, Bismuth, Blue Euclase, Brandenberg Amethyst, Clevelandite, Conichalcite, Cradle of Life (Humankind), Freedom Stone, Frondellite, Green Ridge Quartz, Luxullianite, Nunderite, Nuummite, Shift Crystal, Tangerose. *Chakra:* three-chambered heart

Astrological chart/planetary healers, traditional associations:

Sun: yellowish or gold-coloured stones, Sunstone, Topaz

Moon: whitish stones, Diamond, Quartz, Selenite, Silver

Mercury: neutral or silvery stones, Blue Lace Agate, Rose Quartz

Venus: green stones, copper, Chrysocolla, Emerald, Lapis Lazuli, Sapphire, Turquoise

Mars: stones of reddish hue, Bloodstone, Hematite

Jupiter: blue/purple stones

Saturn: black stones, lead, Galena, Obsidian, Stibnite

Ascendant: Quartz or zodiac sign crystal (see *The Crystal Zodiac*)

And the 'newer' planets

Chiron: Charoite

Uranus: 'neon' hues, Aura Quartzes, Uranophane (use with caution)

Neptune: Aquamarine

Pluto: Malachite, Obsidian, Uranophane

Nodes: Anandalite

Atlantis issues: Ajo Blue Calcite, Atlantasite, Hanksite, Heulandite, Lemurian Seed, Mount Shasta Opal, Picture Jasper, Sacred Scribes

Attachment: Brandenberg, Cradle of Life (Humankind), Drusy Golden Healer, Flint, Hemimorphite, Jasper, Pink Crackle Quartz, Rainbow Mayanite, Tinguaite. *Chakra:* as appropriate

Attachments, remove: Celtic Quartz, Drusy Golden Healer, Flint, Ilmenite, Jasper, Larvikite, Rainbow Mayanite, Shungite, Smoky Amethyst, Stibnite, Tantalite, Tinguaite, and see Spirit release page 374. *Chakra:* or site as appropriate

Attitude, change: Amethyst Spirit Quartz, Axinite, Dream Quartz, Drusy Danburite, Eclipse Stone, Fluorapatite, Heulandite, Lilac Crackle Quartz, Luxullianite, Purpurite, Satyaloka Quartz, Smoky Citrine, Stichtite, Wavellite. *Chakra:* heart or third eye

Aura: Anandalite™, Beryllonite, Golden Healer, Scolecite, Selenite. Hold in front of solar plexus or sweep aura.

Aura, negative patterns embedded in, dissolve: Amber, Amechlorite, Amphibole Quartz, Ancestralite, Arfvedsonite, Bronzite, Cradle of Life (Humankind), Dumortierite, Flint, Garnet in Quartz, Glendonite, Golden Healer, Lakelandite, Nuummite with Novaculite, Rainbow Covellite, Rainbow Mayanite, Scheelite, Spectrolite, Tantalite. 'Comb' over aura.

Aura protect: Amber, Black Tourmaline, Eye of the Storm, Fire Agate, Hackmanite, Honey Phantom Calcite, Labradorite, Mahogany Sheen Obsidian, Master Shamanite, Nunderite, Paraiba Tourmaline, Polychrome Jasper, Sunstone, Tantalite, Tiger's Eye, Turquoise.

Chakra: higher heart or wear continuously

Aura repair after removal of disembodied spirits: Aegerine, Anandalite, Angel's Wing Calcite, Faden Quartz, Laser Quartz, Phantom Quartzes, Quartz, Selenite, Stibnite

Aura, seal: Actinolite, Anandalite, Andean Blue Opal, Brookite, Eye of the Storm, Feather Pyrite, Flint, Galaxyite, Golden Healer, Honey Phantom Calcite, Labradorite, Lorenzenite (Ramsayite), Molybdenite in Quartz, Nunderite, Pyromorphite, Serpentine in Obsidian, Smoky Amethyst, Spectrolite, Tantalite, Thunder Egg, Valentinite and Stibnite, Xenotine

Aura stabilise: Ajo Blue Calcite, Anandalite, Brookite, Ethiopian Opal, Flint, Golden Healer, Granite, Mtrolite, Poppy Jasper, Tantalite, Thunder Egg. *Chakra:* earth star

Auric blockages, remove: Ajo Quartz, Arfvedsonite, Beryllonite, Cradle of Life (Humankind), Fire and Ice Quartz, Flint, Golden Healer, Green Aventurine, Prehnite with Epidote, Rainbow Mayanite, Rhodozite, Serpentine in Obsidian, Strawberry Lemurian. Circle over site.

Auric cleansing: Amechlorite, Anandalite, Black Kyanite, Citrine Spirit Quartz, Fire and Ice Quartz, Flint, Frondellite with Strengite, Golden Healer, Holly Agate, Keyiapo, Lepidocrocite, Mystic Topaz, Nuummite, Phlogopite, Pumice, Pyrite and Sphalerite, Pyrite in Quartz, Rainbow Mayanite, Rutile. 'Comb' aura thoroughly.

Auric cords, remove: Amechlorite, Anandalite, Flint, Lemurian Aquitane Calcite, Nunderite, Nuummite with

Novaculite, Rainbow Mayanite. Circle over site.

Auric energy leakage, guard against: Eudialyte, Eye of the Storm, Gaspeite, Labradorite, Pyrite in Quartz, Quartz with Mica, Spectrolite. *Chakra:* higher heart. Wear constantly.

Auric entities, remove: Amechlorite, Drusy Golden Healer, Flint, Frondellite plus Strengite, Keyiapo, Klinoptilolith, Larvikite, Pyromorphite, Rainbow Mayanite, Selenite Phantom, and see Spirit release page 374. *Chakra:* base, sacral, solar plexus, spleen, third eye

Auric 'holes'/breaks: Aegerine, Anandalite, Brookite, Chinese Red Quartz, Eye of the Storm, Green Ridge Quartz, Labradorite, Lemurian Seed, Scolecite. Place over site.

Auric implants/mental attachments, remove: Amechlorite, Anandalite, Ancestralite, Brandenberg Amethyst, Chinese Red Quartz, Cradle of Life (Humankind), Cryolite, Drusy Golden Healer, Flint, Frondellite with Strengite, Holly Agate, Ilmenite, Klinoptilolith, Lemurian Aquitane Calcite, Lemurian Seed, Molybdenite in Quartz, Rainbow Mayanite, Tantalite, Tinguaite. *Chakra:* third eye. Place on chakra until released, then purify stone immediately.

Authority figures, difficulties with: Ancestralite, Barite, Cradle of Life (Humankind), Freedom Stone, Lakelandite, Pietersite, Pyrophyllite, Sceptre Quartz, Sonora Sunrise. *Chakra:* dantien

Autoimmune diseases, hereditary: Anandalite, Bastnasite, Brandenberg Amethyst, Chinese Red Quartz,

Cradle of Life (Humankind), Diaspore (Zultanite), Gabbro, Golden Healer, Granite, Lakelandite, Mookaite Jasper, Paraiba Tourmaline, Quantum Quattro, Richterite, Rosophia, Shungite, Tangerose, Titanite (Sphene), Winchite. *Chakra:* dantien, higher heart

Autonomic nervous system: Alexandrite, Anglesite, Blue Moonstone, Golden Healer, Merlinite, Tree Agate. *Chakra:* dantien

Autonomy: Candle Quartz, Carnelian, Cradle of Life (Humankind), Faden Quartz, Flint, Freedom Stone, Frondellite with Strengite, Pietersite, Pyrolusite, Pyrophyllite, Rhodolite Garnet, Ussingite. *Chakra:* dantien

– B –

Baggage, releasing emotional: Anandalite, Chrysotile in Serpentine, Cumberlandite, Eclipse Stone, Freedom Stone, Garnet in Quartz, Graphic Smoky Quartz (Zebra Stone), Mount Shasta Opal, Rhodolite Garnet, Rhodonite, Tangerose, Tanzine Aura Quartz, Tremolite, Tugtupite, Wind Fossil Agate, Xenotine. *Chakra:* solar plexus, heart

Balance male/female energies: Alexandrite, Amphibole Quartz, Day and Night Quartz, Khutnohorite, Shiva Lingam. *Chakra:* base and sacral

Balance physical body with etheric: Ajoite, Anandalite, Andara Glass, Astraline, Eye of the Storm, Granite, Larvikite, Nuummite, Rutile with Hematite, Sanda Rosa Azeztulite, Mohawkite, Thompsonite. *Chakra:* dantien

Base chakra: Amber, Azurite, Bastnasite, Black Obsidian, Black Opal, Black Tourmaline, Bloodstone, Candle Quartz, Carnelian, Chinese Red Quartz, Chrysocolla, Cinnabar Jasper, Citrine, Clinohumite, Cuprite, Dragon Stone, Dreamsicle Lemurian, Eye of the Storm (Judy's Jasper), Flint, Fire Agate, Fulgarite, Gabbro, Garnet, Golden Topaz, Harlequin Quartz (Hematite in Quartz), Hematite, Kambaba Jasper, Keyiapo, Limonite, Obsidian, Pink Tourmaline, Poppy Jasper, Realgar and Orpiment, Red Amethyst, Red Calcite, Red Jasper, Red Zincite, Rooster Booster, Ruby, Serpentine, Serpentine in Obsidian, Shungite, Smoky Quartz, Sonora Sunrise, Spinel, Strawberry Lemurian, Strawberry Quartz, Stromatolite, Tangerose, Triplite, Zircon. *Chakra:* place at perineum or base of spine

> **balance and align:** Anandalite, Celestobarite, Green Ridge Quartz, Hematite Quartz, Red Calcite, Red Coral, Ruby, Shiva Lingam
>
> **spin too rapid/stuck open:** Agate, Green Ridge Quartz, Mahogany Obsidian, Pink Tourmaline, Smoky Quartz, Triplite in matrix
>
> **spin too sluggish/stuck closed:** Fire Agate, Hematite, Kundalini Quartz, Red Calcite, Serpentine, Sonora Sunrise, Triplite

Beliefs that no longer serve, release: Ancestralite, Cradle of Life (Humankind), Freedom Stone, Goethite, Lakelandite. *Chakra:* past life, third eye

Betrayal: Golden Healer, Quantum Quattro, Smoky Rose Quartz, Tugtupite. *Chakra:* three-chambered heart

Bigotry, overcome effects of: Chrysanthemum Stone, Rose Quartz, Tugtupite. *Chakra:* heart

Bitterness: Gaspeite, Huebnerite, Rose Quartz. *Chakra:* heart

Blockages from past lives: Ajo Blue Calcite, Ancestralite, Chrysotile, Dumortierite, Flint, Freedom Stone, Lakelandite, Lemurian Seed, Nuummite, Orange Kyanite, Preseli Bluestone, Purple Scapolite, Rainbow Mayanite, Rhodozite, Serpentine in Obsidian. *Chakra:* past life, causal vortex

Blockages, self-imposed: Bowenite (New Jade), Brandenberg, Cradle of Life (Humankind), Elestial Quartz, Freedom Stone, Gold Siberian Quartz, Prehnite with Epidote, Rhodozite, Serpentine in Obsidian,

Sichuan Quartz. *Chakra:* higher heart

Blocked feelings: Frondellite, Indicolite Quartz, Lepidocrocite, Malachite, Mangano Calcite, Montebrasite, Obsidian, Peridot, Pyrite and Sphalerite, Pyrite in Quartz, Rainbow Mayanite, Rhodochrosite, Rhodonite, Rose Quartz, Tantalite, Tanzine Aura Quartz. *Chakra:* three-chambered heart, brow

Blueprint, etheric: Ammolite, Anandalite, Ancestralite, Andescine Labradorite, Astraline, Beryllonite, Black Kyanite, Brandenberg Amethyst, Chlorite Quartz, Cradle of Life (Humankind), Ethiopian Opal, Eye of the Storm, Fulgarite, Golden Healer, Keyiapo, Khutnohorite, Lemurian Aquitane Calcite, Pollucite, Rhodozite, Ruby Lavender Quartz, Sanda Rosa Azeztulite, Scheelite, Seriphos Quartz, Tantalite. *Chakra:* soma, causal vortex

Body:

> **acceptance of:** Candle Quartz, Cradle of Life (Humankind), Eye of the Storm, Flint, Phenacite, Rhodolite Garnet, Vanadinite (make essence by indirect method). *Chakra:* earth, base, crown

> **discomfort at being in:** Candle Quartz, Pearl Spa Dolomite, Quantum Quattro, Strontianite. *Chakra:* earth star, base, sacral, dantien

> **rebalance:** Shiva Lingam, Shungite with Steatite, Victorite. *Chakra:* dantien

> **work efficiently:** Golden Healer Quartz, Phlogopite

Boundaries: Brazilianite, Labradorite, Lemurian Jade, Serpentine in Obsidian, Tantalite. *Chakra:* solar plexus or wear continuously

Break past life/ancestral patterns: Ancestralite, Arfvedsonite, Celadonite, Celtic Quartz, Cradle of Life (Humankind), Freedom Stone, Garnet in Quartz, Green Ridge Quartz, Lemurian Seed, Owyhee Blue Opal, Porphyrite (Chinese Letter Stone), Rainbow Covellite, Rainbow Mayanite, Rhodozite, Scheelite, Stellar Beam Calcite, and see page 352

Broken heart: Cobalto Calcite, Mangano Vesuvianite, Rhodochrosite, Tugtupite. *Chakra:* past life, heart

Bullying: Carnelian, Cat's Eye Quartz, Red Jasper, Shiva Lingam. *Chakra:* dantien or keep in pocket. And see Authority figures page 286, and Autonomy page 287.

– C –

Causal vortex chakra: Ammolite, Anandalite, Ancestralite, Ajoite, Apatite, Azeztulite, Banded White Agate, Black or Blue Moonstone, Blue Kyanite, Brandenberg Amethyst, Celtic Quartz, Cobalto Calcite, Cradle of Life (Humankind), Chrysotile, Cryolite, Crystalline Blue Kyanite, Diamond, Diaspore (Zultanite), Erythrite, Fluorapatite, Freedom Stone, Herderite, Petalite, Phenacite, Phosphosiderite, Pink Flint, Pink Tanzanite, Preseli Bluestone, Rainbow Moonstone, Rhodolite Garnet, Ruby in Kyanite, Ruby in Zoisite, Scolecite, Star Ruby, Sugilite, Tanzanite. Dowse for placement.

> **balance and align:** Anandalite, Blue Kyanite, Brandenberg Amethyst, Celtic Quartz, Chrysotile, Crystalline Blue Kyanite, Fluorapatite, Phenacite, Scolecite, Smoky Elestial Quartz

> **spin too rapid/stuck open:** Black Moonstone, Cobalto Calcite, Diaspore, Flint, Scolecite with Natrolite

> **spin too sluggish/stuck closed:** Ajoite, Blue Moonstone, Erythrite, Herderite, Petalite, Tanzanite

Causes of disease in the karmic or ancestral line, discover: Ammolite, Ancestralite, Chrysotile, Cradle of Life (Humankind), crystal from ancestral or past life locality, Faden Quartz, Golden Healer, Indicolite Quartz, Kambaba Jasper, Lakelandite, Petrified Wood, Pholocomite, Preseli Bluestone, Stromatolite. *Chakra:* past life, causal vortex, earth star

anxiety or fear: Candle Quartz, Dumortierite, Eilat Stone, Khutnohorite, Oceanite, Rose Quartz, Tangerose, Thunder Egg, Tremolite, Tugtupite. *Chakra:* solar plexus, causal vortex, past life

damaged immune system: Ancestralite, Blizzard Stone, Brandenberg Amethyst, Celtic Quartz, Cradle of Life (Humankind), Diaspore (Zultanite), Gabbro, Golden Healer, Lakelandite, Lemurian Jade, Mookaite Jasper, Nzuri Moyo, Ocean Blue Jasper, Pyrite and Sphalerite, Quantum Quattro, Que Sera, Schalenblende, Shungite, Stone of Solidarity, Super 7, Tangerose, Titanite (Sphene), Winchite. *Chakra:* dantien, higher heart, causal vortex, past life

emotional exhaustion from over-caring for family: Candle Quartz, Cradle of Life (Humankind), Golden Healer, Mount Shasta Opal, Prehnite with Epidote, Rose Quartz. *Chakra:* solar plexus

emotional wounds: Ajoite, Bustamite, Cassiterite, Cobalto Calcite, Eilat Stone, Gaia Stone, Golden Healer, Macedonian Opal, Mookaite Jasper, Orange River Quartz, Piemontite, Rathbunite™, Rhodonite, Rose Quartz, Turquoise, Xenotine. *Chakra:* higher heart

mental stress: Candle Quartz, Eye of the Storm, Guinea Fowl Jasper, Lemurian Gold Opal, Richterite, Shungite. *Chakra:* third eye, soma

negative attitudes or emotions: Ancestralite, Candle Quartz, Kornerupine, Pyrite in Quartz, Thunder Egg. *Chakra:* three-chambered heart, crown

past life wounds: Ajo Quartz, Ajoite, Anandalite, Ancestralite, Celtic Quartz, Golden Healer, Green Ridge Quartz, Lakelandite, Lemurian Seed, Macedonian Opal, Mookaite Jasper, Rathbunite™, Rosophia, Scheelite, Xenotine. *Chakra:* past life, causal vortex, earth star

shock, trauma or psychic attack: Apricot Quartz, Black Tourmaline, Empowerite, Golden Healer, Guardian Stone, Linarite, Mohave Turquoise, Mohawkite, Oceanite, Polychrome Jasper, Richterite, Ruby Lavender Quartz, Shungite, Tantalite, Victorite

Celibacy, reverse vow of: Anandalite™, Citrine, Dragon Stone, Freedom Stone, Kundalini Quartz, Serpentine in Obsidian, Shiva Lingam, Smoky Citrine, Triplite. *Chakra:* base, sacral, causal vortex

Cell walls: Ancestralite, Calcite Fairy Stone, Cradle of Life (Humankind), Eye of the Storm, Feather Pyrite, Golden Healer, Poppy Jasper, Shungite, Titanite (Sphene). *Chakra:* dantien, higher heart

Cells: Ancestralite, Celestite, Cradle of Life (Humankind), Dioptase, Garnet, Golden Healer, Herkimer Diamond, Iron Pyrite, Shungite, Staurolite, Yellow Kunzite. *Chakra:* dantien, causal vortex

energetic balance: Golden Healer, Lemurian Gold Opal, Rainbow Covellite, Richterite, Sanda Rosa Azeztulite, Shungite. *Chakra:* dantien

Cellular blueprint: Ajo Quartz, Ajoite, Ancestralite, Brandenberg Amethyst, Chlorite Quartz, Chrysotile, Cradle of Life (Humankind), Eye of the Storm, Fulgarite,

Golden Healer, Kambaba Jasper, Keyiapo, Khutnohorite, Lakelandite, Rainbow Mayanite, Rhodozite, Ruby Lavender Quartz, Scheelite, Seriphos Quartz, Shattuckite, Shungite, Stromatolite, Yellow Kunzite. *Chakra:* higher heart, soma, causal vortex, alta major (base of skull), and see Subtle energy bodies, etheric and karmic page 377

Cellular detoxification: Chlorite Quartz, Eye of the Storm, Fulgarite, Golden Healer, Kambaba Jasper, Klinoptilolith, Larvikite, Rainbow Covellite, Richterite, Seraphinite, Shieldite, Shungite, Smoky Quartz with Aegerine, Stromatolite, Tantalite. *Chakra:* higher heart, causal vortex, alta major

Cellular disorders: Ancestralite, Biotite, Brandenberg Amethyst, Celestite, Dioptase, Eye of the Storm, Garnet, Golden Healer, Herkimer Diamond, Iron Pyrite, Pollucite, Pyrite in Magnesite, Reinerite, Rhodozite, Seraphinite, Shungite, Staurolite, Yellow Kunzite, Zoisite. *Chakra:* higher heart, causal vortex, alta major

Cellular disorganisation: Agnitite, Azotic Topaz, Biotite, Brandenberg Amethyst, Eklogite, Fulgarite, Golden Healer Quartz, Kambaba Jasper, Mangano Vesuvianite, Quantum Quattro, Que Sera, Reinerite, Rosophia, Sanda Rosa Azeztulite, Schalenblende, Shungite, Topaz. *Chakra:* higher heart, causal vortex, alta major

Cellular healing: Ajo Quartz, Ancestralite, Brandenberg Amethyst, Celtic Quartz, Cradle of Life (Humankind), Crystal Cap Amethyst, Elestial Quartz, Eudialyte, Eye of the Storm, Golden Healer, Khutnohorite, Mangano Vesuvianite, Marialite, Nebula Stone, Pyrite in

Magnesite, Rainbow Mayanite, Rainforest Jasper, Reinerite, Rhodozite, Rosophia, Schalenblende, Seraphinite, Shungite, Tantalite, Titanite (Sphene), Zoisite. *Chakra:* higher heart, alta major

Cellular matrix: Ancestralite, Brandenberg Amethyst, Cradle of Life (Humankind), Eye of the Storm, Gold in Quartz, Golden Healer, Kambaba Jasper, Mangano Vesuvianite, Rainbow Mayanite, Rosophia, Shungite, Stromatolite, Terraluminite. *Chakra:* higher heart, alta major

Cellular memory: Ajo Quartz, Ajoite, Ancestralite, Andean Blue Opal, Azotic Topaz, Brandenberg Amethyst, Bustamite, Celtic Quartz, Chrysotile, Cradle of Life (Humankind), Datolite, Dumortierite, Eilat Stone, Elestial Quartz, Eye of the Storm, Golden Healer, Heulandite, Kambaba Jasper, Leopardskin Jasper, Lepidocrocite, Nuummite, Preseli Bluestone, Rainbow Mayanite, Rhodozite, Sichuan Quartz, Smoky Quartz with Aegerine, Sodalite, Spirit Quartz, Stromatolite, Valentinite and Stibnite. *Chakra:* dantien, alta major, causal vortex

Cellular metabolism: Ammolite, Brandenberg Amethyst, Golden Healer, Pyrite in Magnesite, Sardonyx, Shungite, Tangerine Sun Aura Quartz. *Chakra:* higher heart, causal vortex, alta major

Cellular, micro level: Auralite 23, Brandenberg Amethyst, Cradle of Life (Humankind), Dendritic Agate, Fulgarite, Golden Healer, Merlinite, Ruby Lavender Quartz, Seraphinite, Shungite. *Chakra:* higher heart, causal vortex, alta major

Cellular processes: Anandalite, Celtic Quartz, Eye of the Storm, Feather Pyrite, Golden Healer, Shungite. *Chakra:* higher heart, causal vortex, alta major

Cellular regeneration: Ancestralite, Andean Blue Opal, Cradle of Life (Humankind), Elestial Quartz, Eye of the Storm, Golden Healer, Jasper, Kambaba Jasper, Lepidocrocite, Reinerite, Rhodonite, Rosophia, Seraphinite, Shungite, Sodalite, Tantalite, Zoisite. *Chakra:* higher heart, causal vortex, alta major

Cellular repair: Ancestralite, Bixbite, Brandenberg Amethyst, Cradle of Life (Humankind), Glendonite, Golden Healer, Quantum Quattro, Rosophia, Rutilated Quartz, Shungite. *Chakra:* higher heart, causal vortex

Cellular structure: Ajo Quartz, Ajoite, Bornite, Cradle of Life (Humankind), Golden Healer, Hausmannite, Indicolite Tourmaline, Kambaba Jasper, Lilac Quartz, Messina Quartz, Novaculite, Petrified Wood, Reinerite, Rhodozite, Selenite, Shattuckite, Shungite, Stromatolite. *Chakra:* higher heart, causal vortex, alta major

Cellular wall reprogramming: Brandenberg Amethyst, Calcite Fairy Stone, Eye of the Storm, Feather Pyrite, Fulgarite, Golden Healer, Poppy Jasper, Seraphinite, Shattuckite, Shungite, Titanite (Sphene). *Chakra:* dantien, causal vortex

Central nervous system: Anandalite™, Anglesite, Cradle of Life (Humankind), Golden Healer, Larvikite, Merlinite, Natrolite with Scolecite, Prehnite with Epidote. *Chakra:* dantien. Wear continuously.

Chakra attachments, release: Anandalite, Eilat Stone, Flint, Holly Agate, Keyiapo, Klinoptilolith, Larvikite, Lemurian Seed, Novaculite, Pyromorphite, Rainbow Mayanite, Stibnite, and see Spirit release page 374

> **mental influences, detach:** Flint, Novaculite, Nuummite, Rainbow Mayanite

Chakra balance: Anandalite, Auralite 23, Black Kyanite, Citrine, Golden Healer Quartz, Lemurian Seed, Selenite, Sichuan Quartz

Chakra blockages: Ajo Quartz, Amechlorite, Anandalite, Black Kyanite, Chlorite Quartz, Cradle of Life (Humankind), Eye of the Storm, Flint, Fulgarite, Golden Healer Quartz, Larvikite, Lemurian Seed, Picrolite, Prehnite with Epidote, Pyrite and Sphalerite, Rhodozite, Sanda Rosa Azeztulite, Seraphinite, Shungite, Smoky Quartz with Aegerine

Chakra cleanse: Anandalite, Enstatite and Diopside, Flint, Golden Healer Quartz, Graphic Smoky Quartz (Zebra Stone), Novaculite, Nuummite, Orange Kyanite, Rainbow Mayanite, Rhodozaz, Rhodozite, Shungite

Chakra detox: Anandalite, Chlorite Quartz, Eye of the Storm, Flint, Fulgarite, Golden Healer, Larvikite, Pinolith, Seraphinite, Shungite, Smoky Quartz with Aegerine

Chakra energy leakage, prevent: Eudialyte, Gaspeite, Green Aventurine, Labradorite, Pyrite in Quartz, Tantalite, Thunder Egg. *Chakra:* dantien, spleen, solar plexus

Chakra, negative karma, disturbances from:

Dumortierite, Elestial Quartz, Golden Healer, Violane, Wind Fossil Agate. *Chakra:* earth, past life, alta major, causal vortex

Chakras: see also individual names

Chakras, align with physical body: Anandalite, Celestial Quartz, Golden Healer, Keyiapo, Lemurian Jade, Lemurian Seed, Morion, Prasiolite, Preseli Bluestone, Rhodozite, Sichuan Quartz, Sillimanite, Smoky Herkimer Diamond, Thompsonite

Change, facilitate: Celtic Quartz, Cradle of Life (Humankind), Ethiopian Opal, Eudialyte, Fluorapatite, Freedom Stone, Golden Danburite, Heulandite, Luxullianite, Merlinite, Phenacite in Red Feldspar, Quantum Quattro, Scapolite, Shaman Quartz, Snakeskin Pyrite, Tangerine Dream Lemurian. *Chakra:* heart, earth star

Change, ground: Aztee, Basalt, Celtic Quartz, Champagne Aura Quartz, Empowerite, Flint, Fossilised Wood, Kambaba Jasper, Lemurian Jade, Libyan Gold Tektite, Mohawkite, Nunderite, Peanut Wood, Polychrome Jasper, Preseli Bluestone, Schalenblende, Serpentine in Obsidian, Smoky Amethyst, Smoky Herkimer, Smoky Quartz, Stromatolite, Tibetan Black Spot Quartz. *Chakra:* earth star, dantien

Change, psychological: Annabergite, Elestial Quartz, Frondellite, Lilac Crackle Quartz. *Chakra:* causal vortex

Change, vibrational: Anandalite™, Bismuth, Candle Quartz, Celtic Quartz, Ethiopian Opal, Green Ridge Quartz, Lemurian Gold Opal, Sanda Rosa Azeztulite,

Tangerose, Tugtupite with Nuummite. *Chakra:* Gaia gateway, causal vortex, stellar gateway

Chastity, previous vow of: Citrine, Flint, Kundalini Quartz, Menalite, Rhodonite, Shiva Lingam, Smoky Citrine, Triplite. *Chakra*: past life, base, sacral

Childhood, difficult: Anandalite, Cassiterite, Cradle of Life (Humankind), Fenster Quartz, Golden Healer, Pink Carnelian, Red Phantom Quartz, Rhodolite Garnet, Shiva Lingam, Tugtupite, Tugtupite with Nuummite, Voegesite, Youngite. *Chakra:* heart, solar plexus

Chromosome damage: Ancestralite, Brandenberg Amethyst, Cradle of Life (Humankind), Golden Healer, Merlinite, Stromatolite. *Chakra:* dantien, alta major

Chronic dis-ease: Apricot Quartz, Bismuth, Bloodstone, Cathedral Quartz, Golden Healer, Lemurian Jade, Orgonite, Petrified Wood, Quantum Quattro, Que Sera, Shungite, Witches Finger (Magdalena Stone). *Chakra:* dantien

Chronic illness: Apricot Quartz, Bismuth, Bloodstone, Brandenberg Amethyst, Cat's Eye, Cradle of Life (Humankind), Danburite, Dendritic Chalcedony, Diopside, Golden Danburite, Golden Healer, Petrified Wood, Poppy Jasper, Quantum Quattro, Que Sera, Shungite, Trummer Jasper. *Chakra:* earth star, solar plexus, higher heart

Codependency: Bytownite, Dumortierite, Fenster Quartz, Quantum Quattro, Sichuan Quartz, Vera Cruz Amethyst, Xenotine. *Chakra:* base, dantien, causal vortex

Cognitive disorders: Auralite 23, Crystal Cap Amethyst,

Fluorite, Golden Healer, Rhodolite Garnet, Sugilite, and see Mental etc page 341. *Chakra:* alta major

Compassion for oneself and others: Ajoite, Brandenberg Amethyst, Cobalto Calcite, Erythrite, Gaia Stone, Goethite, Golden Healer, Green Diopside, Green Ridge Quartz, Greenlandite, Mangano Vesuvianite, Paraiba Tourmaline, Rhodolite Garnet, Shaman Quartz, Smoky Cathedral Quartz, Starseed Quartz, Tangerose, Tanzanite, Tugtupite. *Chakra:* heart seed

Condescension: Heulandite

Confidence: Candle Quartz, Carnelian, Dumortierite, Erythrite, Eudialyte, Kakortokite, Lazulite, Morion, Prasiolite, Purpurite, Red Jasper, Strontianite. *Chakra:* base, dantien

Conflict resolution: Celtic Quartz, Champagne Aura Quartz, Fluorapatite, Rose Quartz, Shiva Lingam, Trigonic Quartz. *Chakra:* causal vortex

Confusion, disperse: Auralite 23, Blue Scapolite, Celestial Quartz, Crystal Cap Amethyst, Elestial Quartz, Fluorite, Gabbro, Hematoid Calcite, Kakortokite, Lepidocrocite, Limonite, Owyhee Blue Opal, Paraiba Tourmaline, Rhodolite Garnet. *Chakra:* between third eye and soma

Contracts, renegotiate: Anandalite, Ancestralite, Boli Stone, Cradle of Life (Humankind), Dumortierite, Freedom Stone, Gabbro, Nuummite, Prasiolite, Purple Scapolite, Quantum Quattro, Red Amethyst, Shiva Lingam. *Chakra:* past life, alta major, causal vortex

Contraindications and cautions:

Bronzite: Use with caution as it rebounds negative energy back and forth amplifying it. Combine with Black Tourmaline or Smoky Quartz.

catharsis, may induce: Barite, Epidote, Hypersthene, Obsidian, Smoky Spirit Quartz, Tugtupite (replace with Quantum Quattro or Smoky Quartz)

epilepsy: Dumortierite, Goethite, Zircon

giddiness, remove if causes: Banded Agate

heart palpitations, if causes remove: Eilat Stone, Malachite

illusion, may induce: Blue or Rainbow Moonstone

negative energy heightened if worn constantly: Epidote, Hypersthene

psychiatric conditions, paranoia or schizophrenia: Do not use crystals unless under the supervision of a qualified crystal healer.

radioactive: Very dark Smoky Quartz, Uranophane (use under supervision)

toehold in incarnation: avoid Gabbro with Moonstone, Llanite (Llanoite), Polychrome Jasper. *Chakra:* earth star and soma

toxic: The following crystals may contain traces of toxic mineral although these are bound up within the structure (use polished stone, make crystal essence by indirect method, wash hands after handling):

Actinolite, Adamite, Ajoite, Alexandrite, Almandine Garnet, Amazonite, Andaluscite, Aquamarine, Aragonite, Arsenopyrite, Atacamite, Aurichalcite, Axinite, Azurite, Beryl, Beryllium, Biotite (ferrous),

Bixbite, Black Tourmaline, Boji Stones, Bornite, Brazilianite, Brochantite, Bumble Bee Jasper, Cassiterite, Cavansite, Celestite, Cerussite, Cervanite, Chalchantite, Chalcopyrite (Peacock Ore), Chrysoberyl, Chrysocolla, Chrysotile, Cinnabar, Conichalcite, Copper, Covellite, Crocoite, Cryolite, Cuprite, Diopside, Dioptase, Dumortierite, Emerald, Epidote, Fluorite, Galena, Garnet, Garnierite (Falcondoite), Gem Silica, Germanium, Goshenite, Heliodor, Hessonite Garnet, Hiddenite, Iolite, Jadeite, Jamesonite, Kinoite, Klinoptilolith, Kunzite, Kyanite, Labradorite, Lapis Lazuli, Lazurite, Lepidolite, Magnetite, Malachite, Malacholla, Marcasite, Messina Quartz, Mohawkite, Moldavite, Moonstone, Moqui Balls, Morganite, Orpiment, Pargasite, Piemontite, Pietersite, Plancheite, Prehnite, Psilomelane, Pyrite, Pyromorphite, Quantum Quattro, Que Sera, Realgar, Realgar and Orpiment, Renierite, Rhodolite Garnet, Ruby, Sapphire, Serpentine, Smithsonite, Sodalite, Spessartine Garnet, Sphalerite, Spinel, Spodumene, Staurolite, Stibnite, Stilbite, Sugilite, Sulphur, Sunstone, Tanzanite, Tiffany Stone, Tiger's Eye, Topaz, Torbenite, Tourmaline, Tremolite, Turquoise, Uranophane, Uvarovite Garnet, Valentinite, Vanadinite, Variscite, Vesuvianite, Vivianite, Wavellite, Wulfenite, Zircon, Zoisite

Control freak: Chrysotile, Freedom Stone, Ice Quartz, Lazulite, Lemurian Aquitane Calcite, Spider Web Obsidian. *Chakra:* dantien

Core being: Celtic Quartz, Scolecite, Stichtite and Serpentine

Core beliefs: Anthrophyllite, Celtic Quartz, Gabbro, Mohawkite, Tantalite

Core energy: Erythrite, Lemurian Jade, Menalite, Poppy Jasper, Silver Leaf Jasper, Smoky Rose Quartz, Trummer Jasper. *Chakra:* dantien

Core strength/stability: Celtic Quartz, Crinoidal Limestone, Eye of the Storm, Flint, Golden Healer Quartz, Hematite, Mohawkite, Polychrome Jasper, Terraluminite

Country and state stones:

    Africa: Rutilated Quartz, Smoky Quartz

    Alabama: Hematite

    Alaska: Garnet, Jade

    Alberta: Petrified Wood

    Arizona: Sedona Stone, Turquoise

    Arkansas: Ajoite, Quartz

    Atlantis: see page 283

    Australia: Alcheringa Stone, Mookaite Jasper, Opal, Thunder Egg

    Baltic States: Amber

    Bokhara: Lapis Lazuli

    Bolivia: Lapis Lazuli

    Bosnia: Blue Quartz

    California: Mount Shasta Opal, Serpentine, Sonora Sunrise

    Canada: Ammolite, Auralite 23, Canadian Amethyst

    Central and South America: Emerald

Chile: Chilean Lemurian Quartz, Lapis Lazuli

China: Chinese Red Quartz, Jade

Circumpolar regions: Greenlandite, Nuummite, Serpentine, Tugtupite

Colorado: Rhodochrosite

Connecticut: Almandine Garnet, Danburite

Czechoslovakia (former): Garnet

Delaware: Sillimanite

Denmark: Agate

Egypt: Alabaster, Aswan Granite, Black Basalt, Carnelian, Heulandite, Lapis Lazuli, Libyan Gold Tektite, Nubian Golden Healers, Peridot, Turquoise

England: Ammonite, Celestobarite, Diamond, Lakelandite

Florida: Moonstone

France: Amber

Georgia (US): Quartz

Greece: Amethyst

Greenland: Greenlandite, Nuummite, Serpentine, Tugtupite

Hawaii: Black Coral, Peridot

Hungary: Fire Opal

Idaho: Star Garnet

Illinois: Fluorite

India: Himalayan Quartz, Shiva Lingam

Indiana: Limestone

Iowa: Quartz

Iran: Turquoise

Ireland: Snow Quartz

Israel: Bloodstone, Marble, Quantum Quattro, Smoky Quartz

Japan: Chrysanthemum Stone

Kansas: none

Kentucky: Agate

Lemuria: see page 338

Louisiana: Agate

Madagascar: Morganite (Pink Beryl)

Maine: Tourmaline

Maryland: Agate

Massachusetts: Rhodonite

Mesopotamia: Bloodstone, Carnelian, Selenite

Mexico: Emerald, Obsidian, Sonora Sunrise

Michigan: Chlorastrolite

Minnesota: Lake Superior Agate

Mississippi: Petrified Wood

Missouri: Galena

Montana: Agate, Montana Sapphire

Myanmar: Ruby

Nebraska: Agate

Netherlands: Diamond

Nevada: Fire Opal, Turquoise

New England: Tourmaline

New Hampshire: Beryl, Granite, Smoky Quartz

New Jersey: none

New Mexico: Turquoise

New South Wales: Fire Opal

New York: Agate, Herkimer Diamond

New Zealand: Labradorite, Pounamu (Greenstone/

Green Jade)

North Carolina: Emerald, Granite

North Dakota: none

Norway: Carnelian

Ohio: Flint

Oklahoma: Barite Rose (Selenite)

Oregon: Agate, Labradorite, Sunstone

Panama: Agate

Pennsylvania: Celestite

Peru: Emerald, Machu Picchu Stone, Rhodochrosite

Poland: Zincite

Rhode Island: Serpentine

Romania: Amber

Russia: Nuummite, Rhodonite, Sacred Scribe, Shungite

Saudi Arabia: Tektite

Scotland: Cairngorm, Smoky Quartz

Senegal: Rutilated Quartz

Sicily: Amber

South Africa: Ajoite, Diamond, Freedom Stone

South Carolina: Amethyst, Granite

South Dakota: Agate, Rose Quartz

Spain: Aragonite, Emerald

Sweden: Carnelian

Switzerland: Quartz

Tennessee: Agate

Texas: Blue Topaz

Thailand: Ruby

Tibet: Golden Herkimer, Tibetan Quartz

Turkestan: Jade
Turkey: Diaspore, Turquoise
United States: Catlinite, Sapphire
Uruguay: Amber, Uruguayan Amethyst
Utah: Yellow Topaz
Vermont: Granite, Grossular Garnet
Virginia: Nelsonite
Wales: Celtic Quartz, Preseli Bluestone
Washington: Petrified Wood
Wisconsin: Red Granite
West Virginia: Calcedony/Coal
Wyoming: Jade
Place on a map or over appropriate chakras.

Cravings: Amethyst, Auralite 23, Banded Agate, Botswana Agate, Crackled Fire Agate, Freedom Stone, Kiwi Stone, Stichtite, Tantalite. *Chakra:* dantien, solar plexus, and see Addiction page 277

Crisis: Amethyst, Eye of the Storm, Flint, Rhodolite Garnet. Carry at all times.

Crown chakra: Afghanite, Amethyst, Amphibole Quartz, Anandalite, Angelite, Angel's Wing Calcite, Arfvedsonite, Auralite 23, Brandenberg Amethyst, Celestial Quartz, Celtic Quartz, Citrine, Clear Tourmaline, Golden Beryl, Golden Healer, Green Ridge Quartz, Larimar, Lepidolite, Moldavite, Novaculite, Petalite, Phenacite, Purple Jasper, Purple Sapphire, Quartz, Rosophia, Satyamani and Satyaloka Quartz, Selenite, Serpentine, Titanite (Sphene), Trigonic, White Calcite, White Topaz. *Chakra:* top of head

    balance and align: Amethyst, Anandalite, Auralite 23,

Brandenberg Amethyst, Phenacite, Selenite, Sugilite

spin too rapid/stuck open: Amethyst, Amphibole Quartz, Larimar, Petalite, Serpentine, White Calcite

spin too sluggish/stuck closed: Anandalite, Moldavite, Phenacite, Rosophia, Selenite

Curses, break ancestral: Freedom Stone, Nuummite, Purpurite, Quantum Quattro, Shattuckite, Stibnite, Tiger's Eye, Tourmalinated Quartz. *Chakra:* past life, throat, third eye, causal vortex

Curses, deflect effects of: Black Tourmaline, Bronzite (use with caution can rebound), Freedom Stone, Green Ridge Quartz, Master Shamanite, Mohawkite, Purpurite, Quantum Quattro, Tourmalinated Quartz, Tourmaline. *Chakra:* past life, throat, causal vortex

Curses, remove: Aegerine, Black Tourmaline, Flint, Nuummite, Purpurite, Quantum Quattro, Rainbow Mayanite, Shattuckite, Stibnite, Tiger's Eye, Tourmalinated Quartz. *Chakra:* heart, solar plexus, third eye, causal vortex

Curses, turn back: Black Tourmaline, Bronzite (use with caution), Labradorite, Master Shamanite, Mohawkite, Nuummite, Richterite, Tantalite, Tourmalinated Quartz. *Chakra:* throat

– D –

Dantien: Amber, Carnelian, Chinese Red Quartz, Empowerite, Eye of the Storm, Fire Agate, Fire Opal, Golden Herkimer, Green Ridge Quartz, Hematite, Hematoid Calcite, Kambaba Jasper, Kundalini Quartz, Madagascan Red Celestial Quartz, Moonstone, Orange River Quartz, Peanut Wood, Polychrome Jasper, Poppy Jasper, Red Amethyst, Red Jasper, Rhodozite, Rose or Ruby Aura Quartz, Rosophia, Sonora Sunrise, Strawberry Lemurian, Stromatolite, Topaz

> **balance and align:** Empowerite, Eye of the Storm, Green Ridge Quartz, Poppy Jasper
>
> **spin too rapid/stuck open:** Peanut Wood, Polychrome Jasper, Stromatolite
>
> **spin too sluggish/stuck closed:** Fire Agate, Fire Opal, Hematite, Madagascan Red Celestial Quartz, Poppy Jasper, Red Jasper, Sonora Sunrise, Strawberry Lemurian, Triplite

Decision making/overcome indecision: Bytownite, Covellite, Cryolite, Eye of the Storm, Fluorite, Yellow Scapolite. *Chakra:* dantien

De-cursing kit: Tourmalinated Quartz, Nuummite and Novaculite, and see Uncursing page 384

Defensive walls, dismantle: Calcite Fairy Stone, Cradle of Life (Humankind), Rhodochrosite (replace with Interface see page 334)

Degenerative disease: Ammolite, Brandenberg Amethyst, Budd Stone (African Jade), Cradle of Life

(Humankind), Golden Healer, Holly Agate, Nuummite, Scolecite with Natrolite, Stichtite. *Chakra:* dantien, higher heart, causal vortex, alta major

Denial: Tremolite. *Chakra:* heart

Depression: Ajo Blue Calcite, Amber, Amethyst, Ametrine, Apatite, Apophyllite, Botswana Agate, Carnelian, Chrysoprase, Citrine, Clinohumite, Dianite, Eisenkiesel, Eudialyte, Flint, Garnet, Golden Healer, Green Ridge Quartz, Hematite, Idocrase, Jade, Jet, Kunzite, Lapis Lazuli, Lepidolite, Lithium Quartz, Macedonian Opal, Maw Sit Sit, Montebrasite, Moss Agate, Orange Kyanite, Pink Sunstone, Porphyrite (Chinese Letter Stone), Purple Tourmaline, Rainbow Goethite, Rutilated Quartz, Siberian Quartz, Sillimanite, Smoky Quartz, Spessartite Garnet, Spider Web Obsidian, Spinel, Staurolite, Sunstone, Tiger's Eye, Tugtupite, Turquoise. *Chakra*: solar plexus. Wear continuously.

Detoxify body: Amechlorite, Banded Agate, Barite, Chlorite Quartz, Conichalcite, Coprolite, Diaspore (Zultanite), Eye of the Storm, Golden Danburite, Golden Healer, Halite, Hanksite, Hematite, Hypersthene, Jamesonite, Larvikite, Pinolith, Pumice, Rainbow Covellite, Richterite, Seraphinite, Shungite, Smoky Herkimer, Smoky Quartz, Smoky Quartz with Aegerine. *Chakra:* solar plexus, earth star, base

Detoxify emotions: Golden Danburite, Golden Healer, Rhodolite Garnet, Rhodonite, Seraphinite, Spirit Quartz. *Chakra:* solar plexus

Detoxify etheric body: Astraline, Brandenberg

Amethyst, Ethiopian Opal, Eye of the Storm, Frondellite with Strengite, Golden Healer, Lemurian Aquitane Calcite, Pinolith, Rhodolite Garnet, Seriphos Quartz, Shungite, Spirit Quartz, Tantalite. *Chakra:* third eye

Detoxify mind: Auralite 23, Fluorite, Golden Healer, Thunder Egg. *Chakra:* third eye

Detoxify spiritual body: Anandalite, Eye of the Storm, Golden Danburite, Spirit Quartz. *Chakra:* crown

Disconnection from earth: Basalt, Flint, Granite, Hematite, Kambaba Jasper, Moldavite, Lemurian Jade, Libyan Gold Tektite, Picture Jasper, Preseli Bluestone, Smoky Elestial Quartz, Stromatolite, Strontianite. *Chakra:* earth star, Gaia gateway, dantien, soma

Discontent: Covellite, Peridot, Rose Quartz

Dis-ease, karmic causes of: see page 336

Dispossessed: Ancestralite, Apache Tear, Black Onyx, Black Tourmaline, Celtic Golden Healer, Chrysoprase, Garnet, Jasper, Moonstone, Pearl, Petrified Wood, Rutilated Quartz, Septarian, Smoky Quartz, Stromatolite, Unakite. *Chakra:* base and heart

DNA: Ammolite, Ancestralite, Cradle of Life (Humankind), Datolite, Eye of the Storm, Icicle Calcite, Kambaba Jasper, Lakelandite, Petrified Wood, Pyrite in Quartz, Snakeskin Pyrite, Stromatolite. *Chakra:* dantien, higher heart, past life, alta major, causal vortex

DNA, 12 strand: Ammolite, Ancestralite, Cradle of Life (Humankind), Eye of the Storm, Leopardskin Jasper, Petrified Wood, Quantum Quattro

DNA degeneration, reverse: Ancestralite, Cavansite,

Cradle of Life (Humankind), Eye of the Storm, Golden Healer, Natrolite with Scholecite, Petrified Wood, Pyrite in Quartz, Snakeskin Pyrite

DNA, mitochondrial: Ammolite, Ancestralite, Calcite Fairy Stone, Cradle of Life (Humankind), Eye of the Storm, Feather Pyrite, Lakelandite, Menalite, Poppy Jasper, Titanite (Sphene). *Chakra:* dantien

DNA repair: Ancestralite, Brandenberg Amethyst, Cradle of Life (Humankind), Eye of the Storm, Lakelandite, Shungite, Snakeskin Pyrite

Drama Queen: Creedite. *Chakra:* dantien

Dysfunctional patterns, dissolve: Alunite, Arfvedsonite, Celadonite, Dumortierite, Fenster Quartz, Freedom Stone, Garnet in Quartz, Glendonite, Golden Healer, Rainbow Covellite, Rhodolite Garnet, Scheelite, Spider Web Obsidian, Stellar Beam Calcite

– E –

Earth healers: Anandalite, Ancestralite, Aragonite, Black Tourmaline, Brandenberg, Bumble Bee Jasper, Celtic Quartz, Citrine, Clear Quartz, Eye of the Storm (Judy's Jasper), Fire and Ice, Flint, Golden Healer Quartz, Granite, Graphic Smoky Quartz, Halite, Hanksite, Herkimer Diamond, Malachite, Menalite, Picture Jasper, Preseli Bluestone, Purpurite, Rhodochrosite, Rhodozite, Rose Quartz, Selenite, Shiva Lingam, Smoky Elestial Quartz, Smoky Quartz, Spirit Quartz, Tangerine Dream Lemurians, Trigonic Quartz

Earth star chakra: Agnitite™, Boji Stone, Brown Jasper, Celestobarite, Champagne Aura Quartz, Cuprite, Fire Agate, Flint, Galena (wash hands after use, make essence by indirect method), Golden Herkimer, Graphic Smoky Quartz, Hematite, Kambaba Jasper, Lemurian Jade, Limonite, Madagascan Red Celestial Quartz, Mahogany Obsidian, Proustite, Red Amethyst, Rhodonite, Rhodozite, Rosophia, Smoky Elestial Quartz, Smoky Quartz, Stromatolite, Thunder Egg, Tourmaline. Place below feet.

> **balance and align:** Blue Flint, Brown-flash Anandalite, Green Ridge Quartz, Hematite, Smoky Elestial Quartz
>
> **spin too rapid/stuck open:** Flint, Graphic Smoky Quartz, Green Ridge Quartz, Smoky Quartz
>
> **spin too sluggish/stuck closed:** Golden Herkimer, Hematite, Red Amethyst, Rhodozite, Thunder Egg

Eating disorders: Sichuan Quartz, Sugilite, Tibetan Black Spot Quartz

EFT tapping: Amethyst point, Brandenberg Amethyst, Chlorite Quartz point, Citrine point, Clear Quartz point, Rhodolite Garnet, Smoky Quartz point

Egotism: Bixbite, Hematoid Calcite, Lepidocrocite, Rathbunite™, Red Amethyst. *Chakra:* base, dantien

Emotional abuse: Azeztulite with Morganite, Cobalto Calcite, Eilat Stone, Golden Healer, Lazurine, Pink Crackle Quartz, Porcelain Jasper, Proustite, Rhodolite Garnet, Tugtupite. *Chakra:* sacral, heart

Emotional attachments: Aegerine, Ajoite, Drusy Golden Healer, Ilmenite, Novaculite, Nuummite, Pink Lemurian Seed, Rainbow Mayanite, Smoky Amethyst, Stibnite, Tantalite, Tinguaite. *Chakra:* past life, causal vortex, base or sacral

Emotional baggage: Ajoite, Frondellite plus Strengite, Golden Healer Quartz, Porcelain Jasper, Rhodolite Garnet, Rose Elestial Quartz, Tangerose. *Chakra:* solar plexus

Emotional balance: Amblygonite, Dalmatian Stone, Eilat Stone

Emotional black hole: Ajoite, Cobalto Calcite, Quantum Quattro. *Chakra:* higher heart

Emotional blackmail: Tugtupite, and see Tie cutting page 382. *Chakra:* solar plexus

Emotional blockages from past lives: Aegerine, Datolite, Dumortierite, Frondellite plus Strengite, Graphic Smoky Quartz (Zebra Stone), Prehnite with Epidote, Pyrite and

Sphalerite, Quantum Quattro, Rainbow Obsidian, Rhodolite Garnet, Rhodozite, Rose Elestial Quartz, Serpentine in Obsidian, Tugtupite. *Chakra:* past life, three-chambered heart, causal vortex, and see Past life/ancestral healing page 352

Emotional body: Cobalto Calcite, Golden Healer, Mangano Calcite, Oregon Opal, Rhodochrosite

Emotional bondage: Ajoite, Cradle of Life (Humankind), Freedom Stone, Frondellite plus Strengite, Porcelain Jasper, Rhodolite Garnet. Chakra: solar plexus

Emotional bonds in relationships, disconnect: Amblygonite, Brandenberg Amethyst, Cradle of Life (Humankind), Flint, Green Aventurine, Rainbow Mayanite, Shiva Lingam, Stibnite, Tugtupite, Wind Fossil Agate. Chakra: spleen, solar plexus, base and sacral, and see Tie cutting page 382

Emotional bondage: Ajoite, Cradle of Life (Humankind), Freedom Stone, Frondellite plus Strengite, Porcelain Jasper, Rhodolite Garnet. *Chakra:* solar plexus

Emotional catharsis, induce: Barite, Frondellite plus Strengite, Obsidian, Rainbow Obsidian, Serpentine in Obsidian, Tugtupite. *Chakra:* solar plexus (re-stabilise with Apache Tear, Flint, Smoky Quartz or Hematite on earth star)

Emotional conditioning, release: Clevelandite, Drusy Golden Healer, Golden Healer Quartz. *Chakra:* solar plexus, third eye

Emotional debris: Ajoite, Hematite, Pink Lemurian Seed, Rainbow Mayanite, Smoky Elestial Quartz. *Chakra:* solar plexus

Emotional dependency: Cobalto Calcite, and see Tie cutting page 382. *Chakra:* base

Emotional dysfunction: Chinese Red Phantom Quartz, Fenster Quartz, Golden Healer, Orange Kyanite. *Chakra:* higher heart

Emotional equilibrium: Adamite, Merlinite, Porcelain Jasper, Quantum Quattro, Rutile with Hematite, Shungite

Emotional healing: Boli Stone, Cobalto Calcite, Garnet in Quartz, Golden Healer, Mangano Calcite, Mangano Vesuvianite, Mount Shasta Opal, Porphyrite (Chinese Letter Stone), Rhodochrosite, Rhodolite Garnet, Rhodonite, Tangerose, Tugtupite, Xenotine. *Chakra:* three-chambered heart, solar plexus

Emotional hooks, remove: Amblygonite, Cradle of Life (Humankind), Drusy Golden Healer, Flint, Freedom Stone, Goethite, Golden Danburite, Green Aventurine, Klinoptilolith, Novaculite, Nunderite, Nuummite, Orange Kyanite, Pyromorphite, Rainbow Mayanite, Tantalite, Tugtupite. *Chakra:* solar plexus, spleen

Emotional manipulation: Pink Lemurian Seed, Rhodolite Garnet, Tantalite. *Chakra:* sacral, solar plexus, third eye, spleen

Emotional maturation: Alexandrite, Cobalto Calcite

Emotional numbness: Aquamarine, Carnelian, Green Tourmaline, Morganite, Rhodonite, Rose Quartz, Sodalite, and see Depression page 311

Emotional pain: Blue Euclase, Cobalto Calcite, Golden

Healer, Mangano Calcite, Morganite, Morganite with Azeztulite, Rhodochrosite, Rhodonite, Rose Quartz. *Chakra:* past life, heart, higher heart, solar plexus

Emotional pain after separation: Aegerine, Eilat Stone, Golden Healer, Mangano Calcite, Rhodonite, Rose Quartz, Tugtupite. *Chakra:* higher heart

Emotional patterns: Arfvedsonite, Brandenberg Amethyst, Celadonite, Fenster Quartz, Rainbow Covellite, Scheelite. *Chakra:* solar plexus, base

Emotional recovery: Empowerite, Eye of the Storm, Golden Healer, Lilac Quartz, Rhodolite Garnet, Tugtupite. *Chakra:* higher heart

Emotional release: Cobalto Calcite, Golden Healer. *Chakra:* solar plexus, base, sacral

Emotional shut down, release: Ice Quartz

Emotional stability/strength: Mohawkite, Rose Quartz. *Chakra:* base

Emotional tension: Strawberry Quartz. *Chakra:* solar plexus

Emotional toxicity: Ajoite, Arsenopyrite, Banded Agate, Champagne Aura Quartz, Drusy Danburite with Chlorite, Golden Healer, Valentinite and Stibnite

Emotional/ancestral trauma: Ajo Blue Calcite, Ajoite, Ancestral country/state stone (see page 304), Ancestralite, Blue Euclase, Cavansite, Cobalto Calcite, Empowerite, Epidote, Freedom Stone, Gaia Stone, Golden Healer, Graphic Smoky Quartz, Guinea Fowl Jasper, Holly Agate, Kambaba Jasper, Mangano Vesuvianite, Oceanite, Orange River Quartz, Oregon Opal, Peanut Wood,

Petrified Wood, Porcelain Jasper, Ruby Lavender Quartz, Sea Sediment Jasper, Stromatolite, Tantalite, Tugtupite, Victorite. *Chakra:* solar plexus, past life

Emotional turmoil: Cobalto Calcite, Desert Rose, Golden Healer, Mangano Calcite, Porcelain Jasper, Rhodolite Garnet, Rose Quartz. *Chakra:* base

Emotional underlying causes of distress: Eye of the Storm, Gaia Stone, Lemurian Gold Opal, Richterite, Riebekite with Sugilite and Bustamite, Smoky Amethyst. *Chakra:* solar plexus, past life

Emotional wounds: Ajo Quartz, Eudialyte, Fiskenaesset Ruby, Golden Healer, Macedonian Opal, Mangano Calcite, Moldau Quartz, Mookaite Jasper, Prehnite with Epidote, Rathbunite™, Rhodolite Garnet, Rose Quartz, Rosophia, Scheelite, Tangerose, Tugtupite, Xenotine. *Chakra:* past life, heart, higher heart, solar plexus

Emotions, express: Blue Aragonite, Blue Lace Agate, Morganite with Azeztulite, Rhodonite

Entity attachment: see Spirit attachment page 372

Envy, ameliorate: Blood of Isis, Carnelian, Rose Quartz. *Chakra:* solar plexus, heart

Etheric blueprint: Anandalite, Ancestralite, Andescine Labradorite, Angelinite, Astraline, Brandenberg Amethyst, Celtic Golden Healer, Chrysotile, Cradle of Life (Humankind), Elestial Quartz, Ethiopian Opal, Eye of the Storm, Flint, Girasol, Golden Healer, Keyiapo, Khutnohorite, Lemurian Aquitane Calcite, Rhodozite, Ruby Lavender Quartz, Sanda Rosa Azeztulite, Scheelite, Stellar Beam Calcite, Tangerine Dream Lemurian,

Tantalite. *Chakra:* past life

Etheric body, realign/strengthen: Anandalite, Angelinite, Astraline, Ethiopian Opal, Gold in Quartz, Golden Healer Quartz, Golden Selenite, Green Ridge Quartz

Etheric pests: Cryolite, Tantalite, and see Aura page 284

Etheric support: Eye of the Storm, Mohawkite, Tantalite, Tremolite, Winchite

Ethnic conflict: Afghanite, Ancestralite, Azeztulite with Morganite, Catlinite, Champagne Aura Quartz, Chinese Red Quartz, Eye of the Storm, Fluorapatite, Trigonic Quartz, Tugtupite

Everyday reality, difficulty in dealing with: Blue Halite, Bornite, Cathedral Quartz, Dumortierite, Flint, Granite, Lepidocrocite, Marcasite, Neptunite, Pearl Spa Dolomite, Purpurite. *Chakra:* earth star, dantien (or wear continuously)

– F –

Family burdens: Ancestralite, Cradle of Life (Humankind), Golden Healer, Mohawkite, Polychrome Jasper, Rhodolite Garnet, Tinguaite

Family-confidence: Agate, Cat's Eye, Citrine, Garnet, Larimar, Obsidian, Sunstone, and see Positive family beliefs page 356

Family-esteem: Chrysoberyl, Citrine, Hemimorphite, Mangano Calcite, Moss Agate, Opal, Rhodochrosite, Rhodonite, Rose Quartz

Family scapegoat: Ancestralite, Blue Lace Agate, Celtic Chevron Quartz, Celtic Golden Healer, Green Tourmaline, Larimar, Ocean Jasper, Rose Quartz, Scapolite, Tree Agate. *Chakra:* causal vortex, base

Family stress: Ancestralite, Candle Quartz, Chinese Red Quartz, Datolite, Eye of the Storm, Faden Quartz, Fairy Quartz, Glendonite, Golden Healer, Mohave Turquoise, Riebekite with Sugilite and Bustamite, Shaman Quartz, Shungite, Spirit Quartz. *Chakra:* solar plexus, base and sacral

Family ties, strengthen: Ancestralite, Cat's Eye Quartz, Glendonite, Polychrome Jasper, Strontianite. *Chakra:* solar plexus

Fear: Amethyst, Arsenopyrite, Blue Quartz, Cacoxenite, Carolite, Dumortierite, Eilat Stone, Eye of the Storm, Graphic Smoky Quartz (Zebra Stone), Guardian Stone, Hackmanite, Icicle Calcite, Khutnohorite, Leopardskin Jasper, Oceanite, Paraiba Tourmaline, Spectrolite,

Tangerose, Thunder Egg, Tugtupite. *Chakra:* heart, solar plexus

Fear, irrational from past lives: Amethyst, Cradle of Life (Humankind), Eye of the Storm, Revelation Stone

> **of abandonment or rejection:** Clevelandite, Rhodolite Garnet, Rhodozaz, Rose Quartz

> **of death:** Arsenopyrite, Ruby in Kyanite, Ruby in Zoisite, Selenite

> **of dirt and bacteria:** Frondellite, Shungite

> **of failure:** Avalonite, Elestial Quartz

> **of responsibility:** Brazilianite, Hemimorphite, Ocean Jasper, Paraiba Tourmaline, Quantum Quattro

> **of the unknown:** Bastnasite

'Fight or flight': Aventurine, Axinite, Epidote, Eye of the Storm, Gaspeite, Jade, Nunderite, Picrolite, Richterite, Rose Quartz, Shungite, Smithsonite. *Chakra:* base, dantien, solar plexus

> **adrenal overload:** Axinite, Bloodstone, Eye of the Storm, Jade, Richterite

> **balancing:** Chlorite Quartz, Fire Opal, Rose Quartz, Yellow Labradorite

> **calming:** Bloodstone, Cacoxenite, Eye of the Storm, Fire Opal, Green Calcite, Jamesonite, Kyanite, Richterite, Rose Quartz, Tiger's Eye, Yellow Labradorite

Flashbacks: Auralite 23, Black Tourmaline, Celtic Chevron Quartz, Chevron Amethyst, Danburite, Datolite, Flint, Kunzite, Lithium Quartz, Nuummite, Pink Opal, Preseli Bluestone, Rhodonite, Smoky Quartz

Flexibility: Cavansite, Kimberlite

Forgiveness: Diopside, Green Aventurine, Khutnohorite, Mangano Calcite, Rose Quartz, Tugtupite. *Chakra:* higher heart

Frigidity/frozen feelings: Clevelandite, Cradle of Life (Humankind), Diopside, Eilat Stone, Golden Healer, Ice Quartz, Poppy Jasper, Red Jasper, Rhodolite Garnet, Rhodonite, Scolecite, Serpentine, Tugtupite. *Chakra:* sacral, solar plexus, heart, heart seed, higher heart

Frustration, overcome: Chinese Red Quartz, Poppy Jasper, Pyrite in Magnesite. *Chakra:* base, dantien

– G –

Gaia gateway chakra: Apache Tear, Basalt, Bastnasite, Black Actinolite, Black Calcite, Black Flint, Black Kyanite, Black Obsidian, Black Petalite, Black Spinel, Black Spot Herkimer Diamond, Day and Night Quartz, Fire and Ice, Granite, Hematite, Jet, Master Shamanite, Mohawkite, Morion, Naturally Dark Smoky Quartz (not irradiated), Nebula Stone, Nirvana Quartz, Nuummite, Petalite, Preseli Bluestone, Sardonyx, Shungite, Smoky Elestial Quartz, Snowflake Obsidian, Specular Hematite, Spider Web Obsidian, Stromatolite, Tektite, Tibetan Black Spot Quartz, Tourmalinated Quartz, Verdelite. *Chakra:* below feet and/or on stellar gateway

> **balance and align:** Black Flint, Day and Night Quartz, Fire and Ice, Master Shamanite, Morion, Shungite, Tourmalinated Quartz, Verdelite

> **spin too rapid/stuck open:** Apache Tear, Basalt, Black Flint, Black Kyanite, Master Shamanite, Sardonyx, Shungite

> **spin too sluggish/stuck closed:** Black Spot or Golden Herkimer Diamond, Nirvana Quartz, Preseli Bluestone, Shungite, Specular Hematite, Tektite, Tibetan Black Spot Quartz

Genetic disorders: Amblygonite, Ancestralite, Brandenberg Amethyst, Cradle of Life (Humankind), Golden Healer, Kambaba Jasper, Montebrasite, Petrified Wood, Stromatolite, and see DNA page 312. *Chakra:* dantien, solar plexus, alta major, causal vortex

Genocide: Ancestralite, Catlinite, Cradle of Life (Humankind), Freedom Stone, Morion Quartz, Trigonic Quartz. *Chakra:* earth star and Gaia gateway

Grief: Aegerine, Ajo Quartz, Blue Drusy Quartz, Cobalto Calcite, Datolite, Diopside, Empowerite, Epidote, Girasol, Indicolite Quartz, Khutnohorite, Mangano Vesuvianite, Quantum Quattro, Rhodolite Garnet, Rose Quartz, Ruby in Kyanite, Ruby in Zoisite. *Chakra:* higher heart

Grounding: Ajo Quartz, Amphibole, Aztee, Blue Aragonite, Bronzite, Bustamite, Calcite Fairy Stone, Champagne Aura Quartz, Cloudy Quartz, Dalmatian Stone, Empowerite, Flint, Gabbro, Granite, Healer's Gold, Hematite, Hematoid Calcite, Honey Phantom Quartz, Kambaba Jasper, Keyiapo, Lazulite, Lemurian Jade, Lemurian Seed, Leopardskin Serpentine, Libyan Gold Tektite, Limonite, Marcasite, Merlinite, Mohawkite, Novaculite, Nunderite, Peanut Wood, Pearl Spa Dolomite, Petrified Wood, Poppy Jasper, Preseli Bluestone, Purpurite, Pyrite in Magnesite, Quantum Quattro, Rutile with Hematite, Schalenblende, Serpentine in Obsidian, Smoky Elestial Quartz, Smoky Herkimer, Smoky Quartz, Steatite, Stromatolite. *Chakra:* base, earth star, dantien

Guilt: Astrophyllite, Catlinite, Cobalto Calcite, Eudialyte, Hackmanite, Hematoid Calcite, Leopardskin Jasper, Messina Quartz, Pumice, Quantum Quattro, Rhodolite Garnet, Rose Quartz, Steatite, Tugtupite. *Chakra:* solar plexus, higher heart

Guru disconnection: Banded Agate, Rainbow Mayanite.
Chakra: third eye

– H –

Habits, overcome: Heulandite, Oligoclase, Purpurite. *Chakra:* solar plexus

Hearing loss: Alabandite, Ammolite, Budd Stone (African Jade), Kambaba Jasper, Leopardskin Serpentine, Peanut Wood, Smoky Amethyst, Snakeskin Agate, Stromatolite. *Chakra:* past life

Heart, broken: Candle Quartz, Cobalto Calcite, Creedite, Garnet in Granite, Golden Healer, Khutnohorite, Roselite, Ruby in Granite, Ruby in Moonstone, Smoky Rose Quartz, Tugtupite

Heart chakra: Apophyllite, Aventurine, Chrysocolla, Chrysoprase, Cobalto Calcite, Danburite, Eudialyte, Gaia Stone, Green Jasper, Green Quartz, Green Sapphire, Green Siberian Quartz, Green Tourmaline, Hematite Quartz, Herkimer Diamond, Jade, Jadeite, Kunzite, Lavender Quartz, Lepidolite, Malachite, Morganite, Muscovite, Pink Danburite, Pink Petalite, Pink Tourmaline, Pyroxmangite, Red Calcite, Rhodochrosite, Rhodolite Garnet, Rhodonite, Rhodozaz, Rose Quartz, Rubellite Tourmaline, Ruby, Ruby Lavender Quartz, Tugtupite, Variscite, Watermelon Tourmaline

> **balance and align:** Anandalite, Cobalto Calcite, Kunzite, Mangano Calcite, Ruby Lavender Quartz, Watermelon Tourmaline

> **clear heart chakra attachments:** Banded Agate, Mangano Calcite

> **open the three-chambered heart:** Danburite,

Lemurian Aquitane Calcite, Mangano Calcite, Pink Petalite, Pink Tourmaline, Rosophia, Tugtupite

spin too rapid/stuck open: Green Tourmaline, Mangano Calcite, Quartz, Rose Quartz, Tugtupite

spin too sluggish/stuck closed: Calcite, Chohua Jasper, Danburite, Erythrite, Honey Calcite, Lemurian Jade, Pink Lemurian Seed, Red Calcite, Rhodozaz, Rose Quartz, Strawberry Quartz, Tugtupite

Heart, physical: Adamite, Andean Blue Opal, Brandenberg Amethyst, Bustamite, Cacoxenite, Candle Quartz, Fiskenaesset Ruby, Garnet in Quartz, Golden Danburite, Golden Healer, Green Aventurine, Green Diopside, Green Heulandite, Holly Agate, Khutnohorite, Merlinite, Picrolite, Prasiolite, Quantum Quattro, Rose Elestial Quartz, Rose Quartz, Rhodochrosite, Rhodonite, Rosophia, Tugtupite. *Chakra:* heart

Heart seed chakra: Ajo Blue Calcite, Ajoite, Anandalite, Azeztulite, Brandenberg Amethyst, Coral, Danburite, Dianite, Fire Opal, Golden Healer, Green Ridge Quartz, Khutnohorite, Lemurian Calcite, Lilac Quartz, Macedonian Opal, Mangano Calcite, Merkabite Calcite, Pink Opal, Pyroxmangite, Rhodozaz, Roselite, Rosophia, Ruby Lavender Quartz, Scolecite, Selenite, Spirit Quartz, Tugtupite, Violane. Place at base of breastbone.

balance and align: Danburite, Golden Healer, Golden Herkimer, Khutnohorite, Merkabite Calcite

spin too rapid/stuck open: Ajo Blue Calcite, Khutnohorite, Macedonian Opal

spin too sluggish/stuck closed: Fire Opal, Rhodozaz,

Rosophia, Spirit Quartz

Heart trauma: Azeztulite with Morganite, Blue Euclase, Cobalto Calcite, Gaia Stone, Golden Healer, Mangano Vesuvianite, Oceanite, Peanut Wood, Quantum Quattro, Rhodolite Garnet, Rose Elestial Quartz, Roselite, Ruby Lavender Quartz, Tantalite, Victorite

Heart, unblock: Gaspeite, Golden Healer, Mangano Calcite, Pink Lemurian Seed, Prasiolite, Rhodochrosite, Rhodolite Garnet, Rhodonite, Smoky Rose Quartz, Tugtupite

Heartache: Cobalto Calcite, Faden Quartz, Gaspeite, Honey Opal, Pink Crackle Quartz, Pink Lemurian Seed, Morion, Roselite. *Chakra:* higher heart

Heartbeat, irregular: Dumortierite, Golden Healer. *Chakra:* dantien

Helplessness: Actinolite Quartz, Adamite, Brazilianite, Bronzite, Carnelian, Clevelandite, Covellite, Dumortierite, Kakortokite, Mystic Topaz, Ocean Jasper, Paraiba Tourmaline, Pumice, Quantum Quattro, Sceptre Quartz, Tree Agate. *Chakra:* earth star, base, sacral, dantien

Higher heart chakra: Ajo Blue Calcite, Amazonite, Anandalite (Aurora Quartz), Aqua Aura Quartz, Azeztulite, Bloodstone, Celestite, Danburite, Dioptase, Dream Quartz, Eye of the Storm, Fire and Ice Quartz, Gaia Stone, Green Siberian Quartz, Khutnohorite, Kunzite, Lavender Quartz, Lazurine, Lilac Quartz, Macedonian Opal, Mangano Calcite, Muscovite, Nirvana Quartz, Phenacite, Pink Crackle Quartz, Pink Lazurine,

Pink or Lilac Danburite, Pink Petalite, Pyroxmangite, Quantum Quattro, Que Sera, Rainbow Mayanite, Raspberry Aura Quartz, Rhodozaz, Rose Elestial Quartz, Rose Opal, Rose Quartz, Roselite, Rosophia, Ruby Aura Quartz, Ruby Lavender Quartz™, Spirit Quartz, Strawberry Lemurian, Strawberry Quartz, Tangerose, Tugtupite, Turquoise. *Chakra:* higher heart

> **balance and align:** Bloodstone, Eye of the Storm, Quantum Quattro, Que Sera, Tangerose
>
> **spin too rapid/stuck open:** Eye of the Storm, Mangano Calcite, Pink Petalite, Rose Elestial Quartz, Turquoise
>
> **spin too sluggish/stuck closed:** Quantum Quattro, Que Sera, Ruby Aura Quartz, Strawberry Lemurian

Higher Self, contact: Amphibole, Anandalite, Anthrophyllite, Bushman Red Cascade Quartz, Cathedral Quartz, Celestite, Faden Quartz, Fire and Ice Quartz, Golden Healer Quartz, Green Ridge Quartz, Mangano Vesuvianite, Orange River Quartz, Porphyrite (Chinese Letter Stone), Prasiolite, Rosophia, Sugar Blade Quartz, Ussingite

Hippocampus, reset: Apatite, Blue Kyanite, Blue Moonstone, Celtic Chevron Quartz, Chevron Amethyst, Fluorapatite, K2, Magnetite, Nunderite, Porcelain Jasper, Preseli Bluestone, Tremolite, Zircon. Place stone in the hollow halfway up back of skull just above bony ridge.

Home harmonising stones:

> *Grid at new moon:*
>
> **to bring more love into the home:** Cobalto Calcite,

Danburite, Larimar, Mangano Calcite, Pink Tourmaline, Rhodochrosite, Rose Quartz, Selenite

to create *joie de vivre*: Citrine, Green Tourmaline, Poppy Jasper

to create more understanding: Rose Quartz, Tourmaline, Youngite

to create peace and harmony: Eye of the Storm, Larimar, Porcelain Jasper, Selenite

to create well-being and prosperity: Aventurine, Citrine, Goldstone

to encourage everyone to get along with each other: Citrine, Eye of the Storm, Moss Agate

Grid at full moon:

to combat crime or conflict: Sardonyx

to clear negativity: Black Tourmaline, Shungite, Smoky Quartz

to combat crime or conflict: Sardonyx

Homophobia: Chrysanthemum Stone, Oceanite, Zircon

'Hooks', remove: Drusy Golden Healer, Flint, Goethite, Green Aventurine, Klinoptilolith, Nunderite, Orange Kyanite, Pyromorphite, Rainbow Mayanite, Stibnite, Tantalite. *Chakra:* sacral, solar plexus, third eye

Hyperactivity due to effects of past lives: Dianite, Prehnite, Sodalite, Sugilite, Yellow Scapolite. *Chakra*: past life, third eye, causal vortex

Hysteria: Amethyst, Eye of the Storm, Marcasite, Rose Quartz. *Chakra:* solar plexus

Identified patient (takes on the family pain or dis-ease): Cradle of Life (Humankind), Fenster Quartz, Freedom Stone, Golden Healer, Polychrome Jasper

Idleness, overcome: Carnelian, Fire Agate, Poppy Jasper. *Chakra:* base, dantien

Ill-wishing: Black Tourmaline, Crackled Fire Agate, Limonite, Master Shamanite, Mohawkite, Nunderite, Nuummite, Purpurite, Richterite, Tantalite, Tugtupite. *Chakra:* throat. Wear continuously.

Illusions, dispel: Adularia, Fairy Wand Quartz, Ilmenite, Kornerupine, Lemurian Seed, Lepidocrocite, Neptunite, Nirvana Quartz, Quartz with Mica, Vivianite. *Chakra:* third eye

Implants, remove: Ajoite, Amechlorite, Cryolite, Drusy Golden Healer, Flint, Green Aventurine, Holly Agate, Ilmenite, Lemurian Aquitane Calcite, Novaculite, Nuummite, Rainbow Mayanite, Stibnite, Tantalite. *Chakra:* crown or as appropriate

Imposter syndrome: Rhodozaz. *Chakra:* dantien

Impotence: Basalt, Bastnasite, Carnelian, Cinnabar Jasper, Garnet, Kundalini Quartz, Menalite, Morganite, Orange Kyanite, Poppy Jasper, Rhodonite, Shiva Lingam, Sodalite, Triplite, Variscite. *Chakra:* base, sacral, dantien

Inadequacy: Eye of the Storm, Poppy Jasper, Pumice, Rhodolite Garnet. *Chakra:* dantien

Incarnation, ameliorate discomfort in: Ajo Blue Calcite, Celestobarite, Dolomite, Empowerite, Golden Healer,

Guardian Stone, Keyiapo, Moldavite, Orange Kyanite, Peanut Wood, Pearl Spar Flint, Picture Jasper, Polychrome Jasper, Red Celestial Quartz, Riebekite with Sugilite and Bustamite, Rosophia, Sanda Rosa Azeztulite, Snakeskin Agate, Strontianite, Thompsonite. *Chakra:* soma, dantien and earth star

Incest, overcome effects: Cobalto Calcite, Eilat Stone, Golden Healer, Rhodolite Garnet, Tugtupite. *Chakra:* base, sacral, solar plexus (wear continuously, or place over chakras for 20 minutes daily)

Inferiority complex: Pyrite in Magnesite, Rhodolite Garnet. *Chakra:* dantien

Infertility: Banded Agate, Bastnasite, Bixbite, Blue Euclase, Brookite, 'Citrine' Herkimer, Fiskenaesset Ruby, Granite, Menalite, Shiva Lingam, Spirit Quartz, Tugtupite. *Chakra:* sacral

Inhibitions: Poppy Jasper. *Chakra:* base

Injuries, past life: Brandenberg Amethyst, Herkimer Diamond, Onyx. *Chakra:* past life, causal vortex

Insecurity: Leopardskin Jasper, Rhodolite Garnet, Rose Quartz. *Chakra:* base

Institutionalised: Bismuth, Freedom Stone, Golden Healer

Integrity: Porphyrite (Chinese Letter Stone)

Intercellular blockages: Ammolite, Ancestralite, Brandenberg Amethyst, Cradle of Life (Humankind), Gold in Quartz, Golden Healer Quartz, Kambaba Jasper, Petrified Wood, Plancheite, Preseli Bluestone, Pyrite and Sphalerite, Rhodozite, Serpentine in Obsidian,

Stromatolite

Intercellular structures: Ajo Blue Calcite, Ammolite, Ancestralite, Brandenberg Amethyst, Candle Quartz, Cradle of Life (Humankind), Gold in Quartz, Golden Healer Quartz, Lemurian Aquitane Calcite, Messina Quartz, Quantum Quattro, Que Sera, Pollucite, Rhodozite

Interface, create between self and outside world: Andescine Labradorite, Brochantite, Green Aventurine, Green Fluorite, Healer's Gold, Iridescent Pyrite, Jade, Labradorite, Lemurian Jade, Master Shamanite, Mohawkite, Nunderite, Richterite, Scheelite, Serpentine in Obsidian, Spectrolite, Tantalite. *Chakra:* spleen, dantien

Intimacy, lack of: Axinite, Cobalto Calcite, Datolite, Rhodochrosite, Rhodonite, Rose Azeztulite, Rose Quartz, Rosophia, Tugtupite

Intolerance: Pyrite in Magnesite, Rose Quartz

Introspection: Amphibole Quartz, Steatite. *Chakra:* third eye

Irritability: Amethyst, Fluorapatite, Pyrite in Magnesite. *Chakra:* base, sacral, dantien

– J –

Jealousy: Eclipse Stone, Green Aventurine, Heulandite, Mangano Calcite, Peridot, Rainbow Mayanite, Rose Quartz, Rosophia, Tugtupite, Zircon. *Chakra:* heart

Joints: Azurite, Calcite, Calcite Fairy Stone, Cat's Eye Quartz, Cavansite, Dinosaur Bone, Dioptase, Hematite, Kimberlite, Magnetite (Lodestone), Messina Quartz, Peach Selenite, Petrified Wood, Phantom Calcite, Poldervaarite, Prehnite with Epidote, Rhodonite, Rhodozite, Strontianite

Judgementalism: Green Heulandite, Mohawkite, Rose Quartz, Tantalite. *Chakra:* dantien

'Junk DNA', switch on potential: Anandalite, Ancestralite, Azeztulite, Cradle of Life (Humankind), Eye of the Storm, Feather Pyrite, Kambaba Jasper, Poppy Jasper, Rainbow Mayanite, Rhodozite, Stromatolite, Titanite, Trigonic Quartz. *Chakra:* causal vortex, soma, past life, dantien

– K –

Karma, burn off: Ancestralite, Brandenberg Amethyst, Chinese Red Quartz, Cradle of Life (Humankind), Picture Jasper, and see Past life/ancestral healing page 352

Karma of grace, invoke: Anandalite, Ancestralite, Cradle of Life (Humankind), Dumortierite, Freedom Stone, Rose Quartz, Shiva Shell, Sugilite, Wind Fossil Agate

Karmic blueprint: Ancestralite, Chrysotile, Cloudy Quartz, Cradle of Life (Humankind), Dumortierite, Golden Healer, Keyiapo, Khutnohorite, Kyanite, Picture Jasper, Rhodozite, Ruby Lavender Quartz, Sanda Rosa Azeztulite, Scheelite, Titanite (Sphene). *Chakra:* past life, causal vortex, and see Subtle energy bodies page 376

Karmic cleansing: Anandalite, Cloudy Quartz, Cradle of Life (Humankind), Flint, Golden Healer, Holly Agate, Lemurian Seed, Picture Jasper, Wind Fossil Agate

Karmic/ancestral contracts: Boli Stone, Gabbro, Leopardskin Jasper, Red Amethyst, Wind Fossil Agate

Karmic debris: Cradle of Life (Humankind), Golden Healer, Nuummite, Peach Selenite, Rainbow Mayanite, Smoky Spirit Quartz, Wind Fossil Agate. *Chakra:* past life

Karmic debts, release: Flint, Holly Agate, Nuummite, Rose Quartz. *Chakra:* past life

Karmic dis-ease: Covellite, Cradle of Life (Humankind), Golden Healer, Isis Calcite, Kambaba Jasper, Nuummite, Stromatolite, and see Past life, dis-ease page 351. *Chakra:* past life

Karmic/ancestral enmeshment: Ancestralite, Blue Flint,

Flint, Golden Healer, Green Aventurine, Novaculite, Nuummite, Peach Selenite, Rainbow Mayanite, Smoky Elestial Quartz

Karmic wounds: Anandalite, Ajo Quartz, Ajoite, Celtic Quartz, Cradle of Life (Humankind), Dumortierite, Golden Healer, Green Ridge Quartz, Lemurian Seed, Macedonian Opal, Mookaite Jasper, Rathbunite™, Rosophia, Scheelite, Xenotine, and see Past life pages 349–355

– L –

Learning from past lives: Ancestralite, Lakelandite, Muscovite, Peridot, Petrified Wood, Preseli Bluestone. *Chakra*: past life

Lemurian issues: Ajo Blue Calcite, Dreamsicle Lemurian, Healer's Gold, Larimar, Lemurian Blue Calcite, Lemurian Jade, Lemurian Seed, Mount Shasta Opal, Sedona Stone, Selenite, Trigonic Quartz. *Chakras:* causal vortex, alta major, past life, heart seed

Leprosy: Feather Pyrite, Snakeskin Agate

Letting go of past: Axinite, Fenster Quartz, Flint, Fulgarite, Green Diopside, Kakortokite, Kimberlite, Lepidocrocite, Nuummite, Paraiba Tourmaline, Pumice, Scheelite, Zircon. *Chakra:* solar plexus, heart, past life

Limiting patterns of behaviour: Ajoite, Amphibole, Arfvedsonite, Atlantasite, Barite, Botswana Agate, Bronzite, Cassiterite, Celadonite, Chlorite Shaman Quartz, Crackled Fire Agate, Dalmatian Stone, Datolite, Dream Quartz, Dumortierite, Epidote, Garnet in Quartz, Glendonite, Halite, Hanksite, Hematoid Calcite, Honey Phantom Calcite, Indicolite Quartz, Kinoite, Marcasite, Merlinite, Nuummite, Oligoclase, Owyhee Blue Opal, Pearl Spa Dolomite, Porphyrite (Chinese Letter Stone), Quantum Quattro, Rainbow Covellite, Scheelite, Spider Web Obsidian, Stellar Beam Calcite. *Chakra:* base, sacral, dantien, solar plexus, past life

Lost souls: Aegerine, Anandalite, Candle Quartz, Jet Quartz, Rose Quartz, Shattuckite, Smoky Amethyst,

Smoky or Amethyst Brandenberg, Spirit Quartz, Stibnite, Super 7, Trigonic Quartz

Love: Cobalto Calcite, Khutnohorite, Rhodochrosite, Rhodonite, Rose Aura Quartz, Rose Elestial Quartz, Rose Quartz, Selenite, Tugtupite. *Chakra:* heart, heart seed, higher heart

> **accepting:** Mystic Topaz, Tugtupite. *Chakra:* heart, heart seed, higher heart
>
> **compassionate:** Bixbite, Candle Quartz, Mangano Vesuvianite, Rose Quartz, Tugtupite. *Chakra:* heart, heart seed, higher heart
>
> **desperate for:** Pink Halite, Quantum Quattro, Rose Quartz, Tugtupite. *Chakra:* heart, heart seed, higher heart, navel (tummy button)
>
> **fear around:** Avalonite, Rhodolite Garnet, Rose Quartz, Tangerose, Tugtupite. *Chakra:* heart, heart seed, higher heart, navel (tummy button)
>
> **for oneself:** Dumortierite, Eudialyte, Faden Quartz, Gaia Stone, Lepidocrocite, Rose Aura Quartz, Rose Elestial Quartz, Rose Quartz, Tangerose, Titanite (Sphene), Tugtupite. *Chakra:* heart, heart seed, higher heart
>
> **increase capacity to:** Candle Quartz, Strawberry Quartz, Tugtupite
>
> **inner divine:** Anandalite, Candle Quartz, Faden Quartz, Selenite, Strawberry Quartz, Tugtupite. *Chakra:* third eye, crown
>
> **mutual:** Datolite, Green Aventurine, Stellar Beam Calcite, Tugtupite

non-smothering: Botswana Agate. *Chakra:* navel (tummy button)

old, cut the cords of: Banded Agate, Flint, Green Aventurine, Lemurian Aquitane Calcite, Novaculite, Nunderite, Nuummite, Rainbow Mayanite. *Chakra:* solar plexus, sacral, past life, navel (tummy button), spleen

open to possibility of: Mystic Topaz, Quantum Quattro, Rose Elestial Quartz, Tugtupite

tough: Cassiterite. *Chakra:* navel (tummy button)

unconditional: Anandalite, Cobalto Calcite, Crystalline Kyanite, Gaia Stone, Lemurian Seed, Poldervaarite, Rose Aura Quartz, Smoky Rose Quartz, Tangerine Aura, Tiffany Stone, Tugtupite, Zircon. *Chakra:* higher heart

– M –

Matriarchy/mother issues: Jade, Jasper, Menalite, Shiva Lingam, Spirit Quartz. *Chakra:* navel (tummy button), and see Parents

Memory, release suppressed: Revelation Stone

Mental abuse: Apricot Quartz, Golden Healer, Lazurine, Proustite, Rhodolite Garnet, Tugtupite with Nuummite, Yellow Crackle Quartz, Xenotine

Mental agitation: Amethyst, Strawberry Quartz, Youngite

Mental attachments: Aegerine, Banded Agate, Blue Halite, Botswana Agate, Lemurian Seed, Limonite, Pyrolusite, Smoky Amethyst, Yellow Phantom Quartz. *Chakra:* third eye

Mental blockages: Auralite 23, Fluorite, Molybdenite, Rhodozite

Mental clarity: Fluorite, Holly Agate, Merkabite Calcite, Moldau Quartz, Poldervaarite, Realgar and Orpiment, Sacred Scribe, Star Hollandite, Thompsonite

Mental cleansing: Black Kyanite, Blue Quartz, Hungarian Quartz

Mental conditioning, rigid: Drusy Golden Healer, Pholocomite, Rainbow Covellite, and see Patterns page 355. *Chakra:* third eye, crown

Mental confusion: Aegerine, Blue Halite, Blue Quartz, Fluorite, Hematoid Calcite, Limonite, Pholocomite, Poldervaarite, Rhodolite Garnet, Richterite

Mental detox: Amechlorite, Banded Agate, Drusy Quartz

on Sphalerite, Eye of the Storm, Golden Healer, Larvikite, Pinolith, Pyrite in Magnesite, Rainbow Covellite, Richterite, Shungite, Smoky Quartz with Aegerine, Spirit Quartz, Tantalite

Mental dexterity/flexibility, improve: Brucite, Bushman Quartz, Calcite, Coprolite, Fluorite, Green Ridge Quartz, Kimberlite, Limonite, Molybdenite, Seriphos Quartz, Tiffany Stone, Titanite (Sphene). *Chakra:* third eye, crown

Mental dysfunction: Alunite, Star Hollandite, Titanite (Sphene)

Mental focus: Fluorite, Laser Quartz, Sacred Scribe (Russian Lemurian)

Mental imperatives, release: Danburite, Idocrase. *Chakra:* past life

Mental implants: Amechlorite, Blue Halite, Brandenberg Amethyst, Cryolite, Drusy Golden Healer, Holly Agate, Ilmenite, Lemurian Aquitane Calcite, Novaculite, Nuummite, Pholocomite, Tantalite

Mental sabotage: Agrellite, Amphibole, Black Tourmaline, Garnet, Green Tourmaline, Lemurian Aquitane Calcite, Mohawkite, Paraiba Tourmaline, Tantalite, Yellow Scapolite

Mental undue influence, remove: Limonite, Novaculite, Tantalite

Mental upheaval: Eye of the Storm, Guinea Fowl Jasper

Menstruation and menopause problems: Menalite

Miasms: Ancestralite, Cradle of Life (Humankind), Crinoidal Limestone, Flint, Golden Danburite, Golden Healer, Kambaba Jasper, Nuummite, Petrified Wood,

Quantum Quattro, Stromatolite. *Chakra:* earth star, base, past life

Misfit: Rhodolite Garnet, Tremolite. *Chakra:* base, dantien, and see Alienation page 279

Misogyny: Zircon

Multidimensional cellular healing: Ajo Blue Calcite, Ajo Quartz, Anandalite™, Annabergite, Brandenberg Amethyst, Crystal Cap Amethyst, Elestial Quartz, Eudialyte, Fire and Ice Quartz, Fiskenaesset Ruby, Golden Coracalcite, Golden Healer Quartz, Mangano Vesuvianite, Messina Quartz, Pollucite, Que Sera, Rhodozite, Ruby Lavender Quartz

Multidimensional soul healing: Ajo Quartz, Anandalite™, Banded Agate, Celestobarite, Celtic Healer, Eudialyte, Fiskenaesset Ruby, Golden Healer, Halite, Hanksite, Icicle Calcite, Kakortokite, Lemurian Seed, Lilac Quartz, Phantom Quartz, Que Sera, Rutile with Hematite, Sanda Rosa Azeztulite, Satyamani and Satyaloka Quartz, Shaman Quartz, Sichuan Quartz, Spirit Quartz, Tangerine Dream Lemurian, Trigonic Quartz

Multidimensional soul work: Anandalite™, Brandenberg Amethyst, Celtic Healer, Fenster Quartz, Porphyrite (Chinese Letter Stone), Sugar Blade Quartz, Tanzine Aura Quartz, Trigonic Quartz

Multidimensional travel: Afghanite, Anandalite™, Auralite 23, Aztee, Banded Agate, Blue Moonstone, Brandenberg Amethyst, Celestobarite, Golden Selenite, Kinoite, Novaculite, Nunderite, Orange Creedite, Owyhee Blue Opal, Phantom Quartz, Polychrome Jasper,

Preseli Bluestone, Rainbow Moonstone, Sedona Stone, Shaman Quartz, Spectrolite, Spirit Quartz, Stibnite, Tanzanite, Thunder Egg, Titanite (Sphene), Trigonic Quartz, Ussingite, Vivianite, Youngite

Multiple personality disorder: Bastnasite, Brucite

Muscle tension, release: Agate, Amazonite, Apatite, Aventurine, Azurite, Black Obsidian, Blue Moonstone, Blue (Indicolite) Tourmaline, Boji Stone, Brecciated Jasper, Celestite, Dravide (Brown) Tourmaline, Fuchsite, Hematite, Kundalini Quartz, Lapis Lazuli, Magnesite, Magnetite, Malachite, Obsidian, Pearl Spa Dolomite, Poppy Jasper, Selenite, Smoky Quartz, Stilbite, Tiger Iron, Tourmalinated Quartz

– N –

Narrow-mindedness: Kundalini Quartz. *Chakra:* base, higher heart

Navel: Ammolite, Ammonite, Anandalite, Ancestralite, Celtic Healer Quartz, Cradle of Life (Humankind), Flint, Lemurian Seed, Menalite, Preseli Bluestone, Shiva Lingam. Crystals native to the country of ethnic origin.

Necessary change, accept: Axinite, Eclipse Stone, Ethiopian Opal, Luxullianite, Nunderite, Snakeskin Pyrite. *Chakra:* dantien

Negative energy, dispel: Apache Tear, Black Kyanite, Golden Healer, Guardian Stone, Hypersthene, Klinoptilolith, Nuummite, Smoky Elestial Quartz, Smoky Herkimer, Tantalite. *Chakra:* throat, earth star

Negative karma, release: Smoky Elestial Quartz, and see Past life pages 349–355. *Chakra:* past life

Nervous system: Anglesite, Golden Coracalcite, Phantom Calcite

Neural pathways: Dendritic Agate, Golden Coracalcite, Larvikite, Mystic Merlinite, Phantom Calcite, Scolecite, Stichtite

Neurological tissue: Alexandrite, Dendritic Agate, Golden Coracalcite, Golden Healer, Merlinite, Natrolite, Phlogopite, Scolecite

Neurotic patterns: Arfvedsonite, Celadonite, Greenlandite, Porphyrite (Chinese Letter Stone), Rainbow Covellite, Scheelite. *Chakra:* solar plexus

Neurotransmitters: Anglesite, Crystal Cap Amethyst,

Dendritic Agate, Golden Coracalcite, Golden Healer, Kambaba Jasper, Khutnohorite, Merlinite, Ocean Blue Jasper, Phantom Calcite, Que Sera, Scolecite, Shungite, Stromatolite, Tremolite. *Chakra:* alta major (base of skull)

Nightmares: Amethyst, Celestite, Chrysoprase, Dalmatian Stone, Diaspore, Hematite, Jet, Mangano Calcite, Pearl Spa Dolomite, Prehnite, Rose Quartz, Ruby, Smoky Quartz, Sodalite, Spirit Quartz, Tremolite, Turquoise. Place under the pillow or around the bed.

Nurturing, overcome lack of: Amblygonite, Bornite on Silver, Calcite Fairy Stone, Clevelandite, Cobalto Calcite, Drusy Blue Quartz, Flint, Golden Healer, Lazurine, Menalite, Mount Shasta Opal, Ocean Jasper, Prasiolite, Rose Quartz, Ruby Lavender Quartz, Septarian, Super 7, Tree Agate, Tugtupite. *Chakra:* higher heart, base

– O –

Obsession: Ammolite, Auralite 23, Barite, Bytownite, Fenster Quartz, Golden Selenite, K2, Novaculite, Nuummite, Ocean Jasper, Red Amethyst, Spirit Quartz, Tantalite, Vera Cruz Amethyst. *Chakra:* dantien, solar plexus, third eye

Obsessive behaviour: K2, Ocean Jasper, Smoky Rose Quartz, Tantalite

Obsessive-compulsive disorder: Amethyst Herkimer, Fenster Quartz, Flint, K2, Novaculite, Tantalite

Obsessive thoughts: Ammolite, Auralite 23, Azurite, Barite, Bytownite, K2, Optical Calcite, Rhomboid Selenite, Scolecite, Spirit Quartz, Tantalite. *Chakra:* third eye, crown

Oppression: Blizzard Stone

Outworn patterns: Amphibole, Arfvedsonite, Brandenberg Amethyst, Celadonite, Garnet in Quartz, Owyhee Blue Opal, Porphyrite (Chinese Letter Stone), Quantum Quattro, Rainbow Covellite, Rainbow Mayanite, Scheelite, Stibnite. *Chakra:* earth star, base, sacral, solar plexus, third eye

Over-attachment: Drusy Golden Healer, Rainbow Mayanite, Tantalite, Tinguaite. *Chakra:* solar plexus, navel (tummy button)

Over-defended: Honey Opal

Over-dependent: Ussingite

Overexcitability: Dumortierite, Fiskenaesset Ruby

Overreaction: Paraiba Tourmaline

Oversensitive: Paraiba Tourmaline, Proustite, Riebekite with Sugilite and Bustamite, Scolecite, Shungite, Tremolite. *Chakra:* solar plexus

Oversensitive personality: Bastnasite, Hackmanite

Oversensitivity to:

    cold: Barite

    pressure: Avalonite, Pietersite

    temperature changes: Barite, Dinosaur Bone, Luxullianite

    weather: Avalonite, Barite, Golden Pietersite

Overstimulated: Poppy Jasper

Over-thinking: Auralite 23, Bytownite, Creedite, Dalmatian Stone, Rhomboid Selenite. *Chakra:* third eye

Overwhelm: Diopside. *Chakra:* solar plexus

– P –

Painful feelings, assimilate: Cobalto Calcite, Golden Healer, Khutnohorite, Mangano Calcite, Rhodonite, Rose Quartz, Tugtupite. *Chakra:* heart

Palm chakra: Golden Healer, Quartz, Spangolite. *Chakra:* throat, third eye, soma, crown

Panic attacks: Amethyst, Blue-green Smithsonite, Dumortierite, Eye of the Storm, Girasol, Green Phantom Quartz, Green Tourmaline, Kunzite, Serpentine in Obsidian, Tremolite, Turquoise. *Chakra:* heart, higher heart, solar plexus. Keep in pocket and hold when required.

Parents: *Chakras:* dantien, navel (tummy button), base and sacral

> **father:** Citrine, Green Tourmaline, Jasper, Mentor formation, Pietersite, Sunstone
>
> **integrate the inner parents:** Day and Night Quartz, Shiva Lingam.
> And see Matriarchy/mother issues and Patriarchy/father issues
>
> **mother:** Larimar, Menalite, Moonstone, Mother and child formation, Picture Jasper, Rhodochrosite, Rose Quartz, Selenite And see Matriarchy/mother issues and Patriarchy/father issues

Past life: Brandenberg Amethyst, Chrysotile, Nuummite, Oregon Opal, Rhodozite, Trigonic Quartz, Violane

Past life abandonment: Rhodonite

Past life access: Ancestralite, Blue Aventurine,

Brandenberg, Chrysotile, Cradle of Life (Humankind), Dumortierite, Lakelandite, Variscite, Wulfenite

Past life addiction, causes: Amethyst, Iolite

Past life betrayal: Rhodonite

Past life blockages: Lepidolite

Past life chakras: Ammolite, Astraline, Black Moonstone, Blizzard Stone, Blue Moonstone, Brandenberg Amethyst, Catlinite, Chrysotile, Chrysotile in Serpentine, Coprolite, Cradle of Life (Humankind), Cuprite with Chrysocolla, Dinosaur Bone, Dumortierite, Ethiopian Opal, Fire and Ice, Flint, Keyiapo, Lakelandite, Larvikite, Lemurian Aquitane Calcite, Madagascar Quartz, Mystic Merlinite, Oceanite (Blue Onyx), Peanut Wood, Petrified Wood, Preseli Bluestone, Rainbow Mayanite, Rainbow Moonstone, Reinerite, Rhodozite, Rhyolite, Scheelite, Serpentine in Obsidian, Shiva Lingam, Smoky Amethyst, Tangerose, Tantalite, Titanite, Variscite, Violane (Blue Dioptase), Voegesite, Wind Fossil Agate

> **balance and align:** Dumortierite, Picasso Jasper, Rainbow Mayanite, Tangerose, Titanite, Violane (Blue Dioptase)

> **spin too rapid/stuck open:** Black Moonstone, Coprolite, Flint, Petrified Wood, Preseli Bluestone, Scheelite, Sea Sediment Jasper, Tantalite

> **spin too sluggish/stuck closed:** Blizzard Stone, Dragon Stone, Dumortierite, Garnet in Quartz, Rhodozite, Serpentine in Obsidian, Tantalite

Past life/ancestral conflict: Bixbite, Champagne Aura Quartz, Fluorapatite, Nunderite, Purpurite, Rainbow

Mayanite, Trigonic Quartz

Past life/ancestral death, unhealed trauma: Anandalite, Blue Euclase, Brandenberg, Cavansite, Gaia Stone, Golden Healer, Green Aventurine, Green Ridge Quartz, Lemurian Jade, Lemurian Seed, Lilac Smithsonite, Nunderite, Oceanite, Porcelain Jasper, Quantum Quattro, Sea Sediment Jasper, Smoky Brandenberg, Smoky Elestial Quartz, Spirit Quartz, Tantalite, Victorite. *Chakra:* past life, earth star, base, heart

Past life/ancestral debts, recognise: Lemurian Seed, Nuummite, Okenite, Purple Scapolite. *Chakra:* past life, solar plexus

Past life deprivation: Jasper, Prehnite

Past life dis-ease: Celtic Quartz, Dumorterite, Golden Healer, Lemurian Seed, Sichuan Quartz, Tanzanite with Iolite and Danburite. *Chakra:* past life, causal vortex

Past life effect on present: Rhodozite

Past life entity attachment: Chrysotile in Serpentine, Drusy Golden Healer, Green Aventurine, Ilmenite, Larvikite, Lemurian Aquitane Calcite, Novaculite, Nuummite, Pyromorphite, Quantum Quattro, Rainbow Mayanite, Smoky Amethyst, Stibnite, Tantalite, Tinguaite, Tugtupite, Valentinite and Stibnite. *Chakra:* past life, sacral, solar plexus, spleen, third eye

Past life family patterns: Arfvedsonite, Brandenberg Amethyst, Celadonite, Dumortierite, Fenster Quartz, Garnet in Quartz, Polychrome Jasper, Porphyrite (Chinese Letter Stone), Rainbow Covellite, Scheelite, Spirit Quartz. *Chakra:* past life, sacral

Past life/ancestral grief, unhealed: Empowerite, Fire Opal, Golden Healer, Mangano Vesuvianite, Oregon Opal, Rose Quartz, Ruby in Kyanite, Ruby in Zoisite, Spirit Quartz, Tugtupite, Voegesite. *Chakra:* past life, heart

Past life/ancestral healing: Ancestralite, Blizzard Stone, Charoite, Chinese Red Quartz, Cradle of Life (Humankind), Danburite, Dumortierite, Eye of the Storm, Garnet in Quartz, Golden Healer, Infinite Stone, Lakelandite, Lodolite, Merlinite, Obsidian, Okenite, Oregon Opal, Peanut Wood, Picasso Jasper, Pietersite, Rhodonite, Serpentine in Obsidian, Tanzanite, Tibetan Quartz, Tugtupite, Voegesite. *Chakra:* past life

Past life/ancestral heart pain/heartbreak: Ancestralite, Blue Euclase, Brandenberg Amethyst, Cobalto Calcite, Dioptase, Mangano Calcite, Mangano Vesuvianite, Rhodochrosite, Rhodonite, Rose Quartz, Tugtupite. *Chakra:* past life, higher heart

Past life imperatives, release: Ammolite, Lemurian Aquitane Calcite, Novaculite, Nuummite, Tantalite

Past life implants: Amechlorite, Chlorite Quartz, Cryolite, Drusy Golden Healer, Green Aventurine, Holly Agate, Ilmenite, Lemurian Aquitane Calcite, Novaculite, Nuummite, Rainbow Mayanite, Stibnite, Tantalite, Tinguaite

Past life injuries: Flint, Golden Healer, Herkimer Diamond, Onyx. *Chakra:* past life

Past life jealousies: Malachite, Peridot, Rainbow Mayanite, Rhodonite, Rose Quartz

Past life, learning from: Dumortierite, Muscovite, Peridot. *Chakra:* past life

Past life manipulation: Nuummite, Tantalite

Past life memories: Chrysotile, Cradle of Life (Humankind), Dream Quartz, Dumortierite, Preseli Bluestone, Revelation Stone. *Chakra:* past life, third eye

Past life mental imperatives, release: Danburite, Fluorite, Golden Danburite, Golden Healer, Idocrase, Nuummite, Septarian, Tantalite. *Chakra:* past life

Past life misuse of power: Nuummite, Ocean Jasper, Sceptre Quartz, Smoky Lemurian Seed

Past life persecution: Wulfenite

Past life pollutants: Diaspore (Zultanite), Golden Healer, Paraiba Tourmaline, Phlogopite, Pyrite and Sphalerite, Pyromorphite, Shungite

Past life prisoner: Freedom Stone, Idocrase

Past life recall: Amber, Ancestralite, Blue Aventurine, Brandenberg Amethyst, Carnelian, Chrysotile, Dumortierite, Garnet, Lakelandite, Phantom Crystals, Serpentine, Variscite

Past life redress: Charoite, Larimar, Lithium Quartz, Rose Quartz

Past life relationships: Larimar, Lithium Quartz, Rhodonite, Rose Quartz, Smoky Amethyst, Twinflame/Soulmate formation. *Chakra:* past life, base, sacral, heart

Past life rejection: Blue Lace Agate, Cassiterite, Rhodolite Garnet. *Chakra:* past life, heart

Past life resentment: Eclipse Stone, Peridot, Rhodonite, Rose Quartz, Tugtupite. *Chakra:* past life, base

Past life restraint, psychological, emotional or mental: Freedom Stone, Idocrase, Libyan Gold Tektite, Tugtupite. *Chakra:* past life, heart

Past life, sexual problems arising from: Eilat Stone, Kundalini Quartz, Malachite, Menalite, Poppy Jasper, Rutile. *Chakra:* past life, base, sacral

Past life soul agreements, recognition: Brandenberg Amethyst, Green Ridge Quartz, Nuummite, Trigonic Quartz, Wind Fossil Agate, Wulfenite. *Chakra:* past life, higher crown

Past life, soul loss resulting from: Chrysotile in Serpentine, Fulgarite

Past life tie cutting: Flint, Green Aventurine, Green Obsidian, Malachite, Novaculite, Nuummite, Petalite, Rainbow Mayanite, Rainbow Obsidian, Smoky Amethyst, Sunstone, Wulfenite. *Chakra:* past life, base, sacral, solar plexus, third eye

Past life thought forms, release: Aegerine, Auralite 23, Iolite, Pyromorphite, Scolecite, Septarian, Spectrolite, Xenotine. *Chakra:* past life, third eye

Past life trauma: Anandalite, Blue Euclase, Brandenberg Amethyst, Dumortierite, Empowerite, Golden Healer, Mangano Vesuvianite, Oceanite, Oregon Opal, Phantom Crystals, Red Phantom Quartz, Ruby Lavender Quartz, Selenite, Smoky Elestial Quartz, Smoky Herkimer, Tantalite, Victorite

Past life vows: Blue Aventurine, Nuummite, Rainbow Mayanite, Stibnite, Wind Fossil Agate. *Chakra:* past life, third eye

Past life vows, release: Andean Opal, Dumortierite, Libyan Gold Tektite, Nuummite, Rainbow Mayanite, Turquoise. *Chakra:* past life

Past life wound imprints in etheric body: Ajo Quartz, Anandalite, Ancestralite, Brandenberg Amethyst, Charoite, Diaspore (Zultanite), Ethiopian Opal, Eye of the Storm, Flint, Golden Healer, Green Ridge Quartz, Lemurian Aquitane Calcite, Lemurian Seed, Macedonian Opal, Master Shamanite, Mookaite Jasper, Rainbow Mayanite, Sceptre Quartz, Selenite, Smoky Quartz, Snakeskin Pyrite, Stibnite, Tantalite, Tibetan Black Spot Quartz. *Chakra:* past life, causal vortex or place over site

Past lives, access: Brandenberg Amethyst, Cavansite, Chrysotile, Cradle of Life (Humankind), Dream Quartz, Dumortierite, Faden Quartz, Fiskenaesset Ruby, Lemurian Seed, Nuummite, Oregon Opal, Picture Jasper, Preseli Bluestone, Trigonic Quartz. *Chakra:* past life, third eye, causal vortex

Past, release from: Dumortierite, Elestial Quartz, Smoky Amethyst, and see Past lives above. *Chakra:* past life, earth star, base

Patriarchy/father issues: Flint, Galena (wash hands after use, make essence by indirect method), Petrified Wood, Shiva Lingam, Smoky Quartz, Stibnite, Sunstone. *Chakra:* dantien, sacral, and see Parents

Patterns, dissolve: Brandenberg Amethyst, Danburite, Flint, Golden Danburite, Golden Healer, Idocrase, Nuummite, Septarian, Stibnite, Tantalite

People-pleaser: Anthrophyllite. *Chakra:* dantien

Persecution: Aragonite, Rose Quartz, Wulfenite. *Chakra:* past life

Personal power, regain: Basalt, Brandenberg Amethyst, Conichalcite, Empowerite, Eudialyte, Eye of the Storm, Kundalini Quartz, Orange Kyanite, Owyhee Blue Opal, Sceptre Quartz, Sedona Stone, Shungite, Tinguaite, Triplite. *Chakra:* base, dantien

Phobias: Amethyst, Andean Blue Opal, Dumortierite, Emerald, Frondellite with Strengite, Girasol, Hackmanite, Heulandite, Oceanite, Prehnite. *Chakra:* past life, solar plexus, base

> **resulting from past life events:** Amethyst, Carnelian, Carolite, Dumortierite, Golden Healer, Oceanite, Prehnite, Serpentine in Obsidian. *Chakra:* past life

Pomposity: Kiwi Stone, Territulla Agate, Youngite

'Poor me' syndrome: Lemurian Jade

Positive family beliefs:

> **Assertiveness is OK:** Carnelian, Jasper

> **Family-acceptance:** Charoite, Jade, Larimar, Mangano Calcite

> **Honesty with each other is OK:** Angelite, Blue Lace Agate, Jasper, Lapis Lazuli, Sodalite, Topaz

> **It's OK to grow up and become independent:** Agate, Emerald, Malachite, Sunstone

> **It's OK to set boundaries – and to challenge them:** Banded Agate, Malachite, Rhodonite, Stromatolite

> **It's OK to shine and be special:** Citrine, Orange Calcite, Sunstone, Topaz

> **Open communication is OK:** Angelite, Blue Lace

Agate, Blue Tourmaline, Kunzite, Sodalite

Risk-taking is OK: Aquamarine, Carnelian, Eye of the Storm, Malachite

We deal with things constructively: Jasper

We learn by our mistakes: Blue Aventurine, Peridot

We love each other no matter what: Chalcedony, Chrysocolla, Mangano Calcite, Pink Agate, Rhodochrosite, Rose Quartz

We trust each other: Amazonite, Blue Quartz, Chrysanthemum Stone, Chrysoprase, Dalmatian Stone, Green Aventurine, Kunzite, Mangano Calcite, Pink Smithsonite, Rose Quartz, Sodalite, Turquoise

We value self-worth and equality: Chrysoberyl, Dalmatian Stone, Larimar, Mangano Calcite, Tiger's Eye

We're OK: Lapis Lazuli, Rose Quartz, Sodalite

Post-Traumatic Stress disorder: see PTSD

Power, overcome misuse of: Nuummite, Sceptre Quartz, Shungite with Steatite, Smoky Lemurian. *Chakra:* past life, base

Premature ejaculation: Hematite, Menalite, Poppy Jasper (brown shades), Rutile. *Chakra:* base and sacral

Prisoner, past-life: Freedom Stone, Idocrase. *Chakra*: past life, base

Prohibitions on using psychic sight: Apophyllite pyramid, Aquamarine, Astrophyllite, Azurite, Bytownite, Lapis Lazuli, Rhomboid Selenite. *Chakra:* third eye

Psoas muscle, release: see Muscle tension, release page

Psychic blockages: Afghanite, Ajo Quartz, Blue Selenite, Bytownite, Rhodozite, Rhomboid Selenite. *Chakra:* third eye

Psychic implants/imprints: Amechlorite, Brandenberg Amethyst, Cryolite, Drusy Golden Healer, Ethiopian Opal, Flint, Holly Agate, Ilmenite, Lemurian Aquitane Calcite, Novaculite, Nuummite, Pyromorphite, Rainbow Mayanite, Snakeskin Pyrite, Stichtite, Tantalite

Psychic interference: Afghanite, Black Tourmaline, Master Shamanite, Nuummite, Purpurite, Rainbow Mayanite, Shungite, Tantalite

Psychic manipulation: Banded Agate, Nuummite

Psychic overwhelm: Healer's Gold, Labradorite, Limonite, Master Shamanite

Psychic shield: Actinolite, Amphibole, Azotic Topaz, Aztee, Black Tourmaline, Bornite, Bowenite (New Jade), Brandenberg Amethyst, Brazilianite, Celestobarite, Chlorite Shaman Quartz, Crackled Fire Agate, Fiskenaesset Ruby, Frondellite with Strengite, Gabbro, Graphic Smoky Quartz (Zebra Stone), Hanksite, Iridescent Pyrite, Keyiapo, Labradorite, Lorenzenite (Ramsayite), Marcasite, Master Shamanite, Mohave Turquoise, Mohawkite, Owyhee Blue Opal, Polychrome Jasper, Purpurite, Pyromorphite, Quantum Quattro, Red Amethyst, Silver Leaf Jasper, Smoky Amethyst, Smoky Elestial Quartz, Tantalite, Thunder Egg, Valentinite and Stibnite, Xenotine

Psychic trauma: Blue Euclase, Empowerite, Eye of the

Storm, Lemurian Seed, Mangano Vesuvianite, Morion, Oceanite, Ruby Lavender Quartz, Smoky Lemurian Seed, Tangerine Aura Quartz, Tantalite, Victorite

Psychic vampirism: Actinolite, Ammolite, Apple Aura Quartz, Banded Agate, Black Tourmaline, Gaspeite, Green Aventurine, Iridescent Pyrite, Jade, Labradorite, Lemurian Aquitane Calcite, Nunderite, Prasiolite, Tantalite, Xenotine

Psychological autonomy, find: Pyrophyllite, Xenotine. *Chakra:* dantien

Psychological balance, gain: Amblygonite, Auralite 23, Fluorite

Psychological catharsis, mediate: Barite, Epidote, Eye of the Storm, Gaia Stone, Nirvana Quartz, Smoky Elestial Quartz, Smoky Spirit Quartz

Psychological healing: Agrellite, Ajoite, Annabergite, Black Kyanite, Diopside, Flint, Fulgarite, Golden Healer, Lemurian Jade, Lemurian Seed, Nuummite, Ocean Jasper, Quantum Quattro, Smoky Elestial, Stellar Beam Calcite

Psychological insights: Actinolite, Lazulite, Leopardskin Serpentine, Septarian, Shiva Lingam, Smoky Brandenberg Amethyst

Psychological integration: Graphic Smoky Quartz (Zebra Stone), Zircon

Psychological shadow: Agrellite, Azeztulite with Morganite, Champagne Aura Quartz, Covellite, Day and Night Quartz, Lazulite, Lemurian Seed, Molybdenite, Nuummite, Phantom Quartz, Proustite, Shaman Quartz,

Smoky Elestial Quartz, Voegesite. *Chakra:* solar plexus

Psychosexual problems: Cobalto Calcite, Dumortierite, Eilat Stone, Malachite (use as polished stone, make remedy by indirect method), Serpentine in Obsidian, Shiva Lingam, Triplite. *Chakra:* past life, base, sacral, soma.

Psychosomatic disease: Andescine Labradorite, Angel's Wing Calcite, Astraline, Azeztulite with Morganite, Azotic Topaz, Benitoite, Dumortierite, Fire Obsidian, Gaia Stone, Golden Danburite, Golden Healer, Icicle Calcite, Larvikite, Ocean Blue Jasper, Roselite, Snakeskin Pyrite, Titanite (Sphene), Voegesite. *Chakra:* third eye, higher heart

> **from sexual abuse:** Azeztulite with Morganite, Golden Healer, Menalite, Shiva Lingam
>
> **understand causes of:** Azotic Topaz, Benitoite, Chalcopyrite, Faden Quartz, Icicle Calcite, Kornerupine, Stichtite and Serpentine, Voegesite

PTSD: Agate, Amethyst, Anandalite, Ancestralite, Auralite 23, Aventurine, Azurite, Bird's Eye Jasper, Black Tourmaline, Blue Kyanite, Brandenberg Amethyst, Citrine, Cradle of Life (Humankind), Danburite, Eisenkiesel, Empowerite, Eye of the Storm (Judy's Jasper), Flint, Garnet, Green Andalucite, Green Calcite, Green Fluorite, Hematite, Hiddenite (Green Kunzite), Kunzite, Lakelandite, Lapis Lazuli, Lepidolite, Mangano Calcite, Nuummite, Onyx, Preseli Bluestone, Red Tiger's Eye, Rhodochrosite, Richterite, Rose Quartz, Rutilated Quartz, Selenite, Shiva Lingam, Shiva Shell, Shungite,

Tangerine Aura Quartz, Tangerine Dream Lemurian, Tangerine Quartz, Victorite. *Chakras:* earth, base, dantien, solar plexus, higher heart, third eye, causal vortex, past life. Wear continuously or grid around the bed, and see page 99 for healing layout.

– Q –

Qi, depleted ancestral line: Ammolite, Budd Stone (African Jade), Chalcopyrite, Eye of the Storm (Judy's Jasper), Golden Healer, Granite, Poppy Jasper, Que Sera, Rhodozite, Ruby in Granite, Sonora Sunrise, Triplite, Violane, Witches Finger/Magdalena Stone. *Chakra:* sacral, dantien

Quick fix: Amethyst, Anandalite, Ancestralite, Boji Stones, Dumortierite, Eye of the Storm, Flint, Golden Healer, Hematite, Labradorite, Shungite

– R –

Racism: Catlinite, Freedom Stone, Zircon

Recall the past: Amber, Carnelian, Chrysotile, Dumortierite, Garnet, Phantom Crystals, Serpentine, Variscite. *Chakra*: past life, brow, and see Reading the Akashic Record, page 178

Reclaim power: Brandenberg Amethyst, Eilat Stone, Empowerite, Leopardskin Jasper, Nuummite, Owyhee Blue Opal, Rainbow Mayanite, Sceptre Quartz, Shiva Lingam, Smoky Elestial Quartz, Tinguaite. *Chakra:* past life, base

Reconciliation: Afghanite, Chinese Red Quartz, Pink Lazurine, Rose Quartz, Ruby Lavender Quartz. *Chakra:* heart seed

Redress the past: Charoite. *Chakra*: past life

Regression: Blue Aventurine, Brandenberg Amethyst, Celtic Quartz, Chrysotile, Dumortierite, Flint, Lakelandite, Kambaba Jasper, Lakelandite, Lemurian Seed, Petrified Wood, Preseli Bluestone, Stromatolite, Variscite, Wind Fossil Agate. *Chakra*: past life, brow

Reiki: Anandalite, Black Jasper, Calcite, Citrine, Lepidolite, Mangano Calcite, Moonstone, Quartz, Quantum Quattro, Rose Quartz, Smoky Quartz, Turquoise, and see entries for crystals that harmonise with the various chakras

Rejection: Blue Lace Agate, Charoite, Rhodochrosite, Rose Quartz, Selenite. *Chakra*: past life, heart

Release anger and tension: Alabaster, Blue Phantom

Quartz, Chinese Red Quartz, Cinnabar in Jasper, Ethiopian Opal, Greenlandite, Nzuri Moyo, Pearl Spa Dolomite, Phosphosiderite, Tugtupite, Ussingite. *Chakra:* base, dantien

Release vows: Banded Agate, Brandenberg Amethyst, Dumortierite, Green Aventurine, Stibnite, Turquoise. *Chakra*: past life, brow

Repressed anger: Cinnabar in Jasper, Ethiopian Opal, Nzuri Moyo, Phosphosiderite. *Chakra:* base, dantien

Repressed emotions: Ethiopian Opal, Golden Healer, Morganite with Azeztulite

Resentment: Eclipse Stone, Eudialyte, Rhodonite. *Chakra:* base, dantien, past life

Resistance to change: Dragon Stone, Eclipse Stone, Luxullianite, Montebrasite, Snakeskin Pyrite, Tangerose. *Chakra*: base, dantien, heart

Restore trust: Clevelandite, Faden Quartz, Rhodolite Garnet, Xenotine

Restraint, emotional or mental: Idocrase. Chakra: past life, heart

Retrieval, child or soul parts: Anandalite, Fulgarite, Khutnohorite, Pink Carnelian, Tangerose, Youngite. *Chakra:* causal vortex, past life

Retrieve soul parts left at previous death: Lemurian Seed, Selenite, Smoky Spirit Quartz. *Chakra:* causal vortex, past life

RNA stabilising: Ancestralite, Chalcopyrite, Kambaba Jasper, Petrified Wood, Stromatolite. *Chakra:* dantien

– S –

Sabotage, self: Agrellite, Amphibole, Black Tourmaline, Blue Scapolite, Garnet, Green Tourmaline, Lemurian Aquitane Calcite, Mohawkite, Paraiba Tourmaline, Scheelite, Tantalite

Sacral chakra: Amber, Amphibole, Apricot Quartz, Bastnasite, Black Opal, Blue Jasper, Blue-green Fluorite, Blue-green Turquoise, Bumble Bee Jasper, Carnelian, Chinese Red Quartz, Citrine, Clinohumite, Golden and iron-coated Green Ridge Quartz, Golden Healer Quartz, Keyiapo, Limonite, Mahogany Obsidian, Orange Calcite, Orange Carnelian, Orange Kyanite, Orange Zincite, Realgar and Orpiment, Red Amethyst, Red Jasper, Red/Orange Zincite, Tangerine Dream Lemurian, Tangerose, Topaz, Triplite, Vanadinite (make essence by indirect method). *Chakra:* sacral/navel

  balance and align: Anandalite, Celestobarite, Golden Healer Quartz, Green Ridge Quartz

  spin too rapid/stuck open: Amber, Black Opal, Blue-green Fluorite, Blue-green Turquoise

  spin too sluggish/stuck closed: Carnelian, Orange Zincite, Topaz, Triplite

Sadness, release: Indicolite Quartz, Rose Quartz, Ruby in Kyanite, Ruby in Zoisite, Sugilite. *Chakra:* solar plexus, heart

Saviour complex: Cassiterite

Scapegoating behaviour: Champagne Aura Quartz, Mohawkite, Scapolite, Smoky Amethyst, and see Family scapegoat page 321

Secrets, keep safe: Nunderite

Security issues: Chinese Red Quartz, Nzuri Moyo. *Chakra:* base

> **emotional:** Mangano Vesuvianite, Oceanite, Tugtupite. *Chakra:* base, dantien, solar plexus

> **letting go of:** Axinite, Scheelite. *Chakra:* base, dantien

Self-acceptance: Lavender Quartz, Lemurian Seed, Orange Phantom, Peach Selenite, Quantum Quattro, Rhodolite Garnet, Tangerose, Tugtupite. *Chakra:* heart, higher heart

Self-awareness: Citrine Spirit Quartz

Self-confidence: Blue Quartz, Lemurian Seed, Nunderite, Pink Sunstone

Self-criticism: Epidote

Self-deception: Nunderite, Oregon Opal

Self-defeating programs: Desert Rose, Drusy Quartz, Kinoite, Nuummite, Paraiba Tourmaline, Quantum Quattro, Strawberry Quartz

Self-discipline: Blue Quartz, Dumortierite, Scapolite, Sillimanite

Self-doubt: Rosophia

Self-esteem: Eisenkiesel, Graphic Smoky Quartz (Zebra Stone), Hackmanite, Lazulite, Morion, Nzuri Moyo, Pink Phantom, Strawberry Quartz, Tinguaite. *Chakra:* base, sacral, dantien, heart, higher heart

Self-expression: Blue Lace Agate, Eilat Stone, Mariposite, Owyhee Blue Opal. *Chakra:* throat

Self-forgiveness: Chinese Red Quartz, Eudialyte,

Luvulite, Pink Crackle Quartz, Rose Quartz, Spirit Quartz, Steatite, Tugtupite

Self-hatred (combating): Blizzard Stone, Luvulite, Quantum Quattro, Rose Quartz, Spirit Quartz, Sugilite, Tugtupite. *Chakra:* base

Self-healing: Benitoite, Elestial Quartz, Eudialyte, Faden Quartz, Gaia Stone, Golden Healer, Morion, Quantum Quattro, Rosophia, Septarian

Self-image, poor: Dianite, Kinoite, Trummer Jasper

Self-nurturing: Poppy Jasper, Porcelain Jasper, Quantum Quattro, Septarian, Smoky Cathedral Quartz, Super 7

Self-pity: Epidote

Self-preservation: Dumortierite

Self-respect: Rainforest Jasper

Self-sabotaging behaviour: Agrellite, Quantum Quattro, Scapolite

Self-sufficiency: Nunderite, Quantum Quattro. *Chakra:* base

Self-trust: Honey Calcite. *Chakra:* sacral

Self-worth: Rhodolite Garnet, Rose Aura Quartz. *Chakra:* base, sacral

Sense of belonging: Polychrome Jasper. *Chakra:* earth star and base

Sexual abuse: Apricot Quartz, Azeztulite with Morganite, Eilat Stone, Golden Healer, Honey Opal, Lazurine, Orange Kyanite, Pink Crackle Quartz, Proustite, Rhodochrosite, Rhodolite Garnet, Rhodonite, Shiva Lingam, Tugtupite, Xenotine. *Chakra:* base, sacral, dantien

Sexual problems arising from past events: Malachite (use as polished stone, make remedy by indirect method), Morganite with Azeztulite, Rhodonite, Rose Quartz. *Chakra:* past life, base, sacral

Shadow, integrate: Morion, Proustite, Smoky Lemurian Seed, Voegesite

Shame: Azeztulite with Morganite, Catlinite, Luvulite, Rhodolite Garnet, Rose Quartz. *Chakra:* base, dantien

Slavery, release from: Apache Tear, Freedom Stone, Malachite, Rainbow Obsidian, Rutilated Quartz

Solar plexus chakra: Calcite, Citrine, Citrine Herkimer, Golden Azeztulite, Golden Beryl, Golden Calcite, Golden Coracalcite, Golden Danburite, Golden Enhydro, Golden Healer, Golden Labradorite (Bytownite), Green Chrysoprase, Green Prehnite, Green Ridge Quartz, Jasper, Libyan Glass Tektite, Light Green Hiddenite, Malachite (use as polished stone, make essence by indirect method), Obsidian, Rainbow Obsidian, Rhodochrosite, Rhodozite, Smoky Quartz, Sunstone, Tangerine Aura Quartz, Tangerine Dream Lemurian Seed, Tiger's Eye, Yellow Tourmaline, Yellow Zincite

> **balance and align:** Anandalite, Citrine, Lemurian Seed
>
> **spin too rapid/stuck open:** Calcite, Light Green Hiddenite, Malachite, Rainbow Obsidian, Smoky Quartz
>
> **spin too sluggish/stuck closed:** Golden Calcite, Golden Danburite, Tangerine Aura Quartz, Yellow Labradorite (Bytownite)

Soma chakra: Afghanite, Amechlorite, Angelinite, Angel's Wing Calcite, Astraline, Auralite 23, Azeztulite, Banded Agate, Brandenberg Amethyst, Champagne Aura Quartz, Crystal Cap Amethyst, Diaspore (Zultanite), Faden Quartz, Fire and Ice, Holly Agate, Ilmenite, Isis Calcite, Lemurian Aquitane Calcite, Merkabite Calcite, Natrolite, Nuummite, Owyhee Blue Opal, Pentagonite, Petalite, Phantom Calcite, Phenacite on Fluorite, Preseli Bluestone, Red Amethyst, Sacred Scribe, Satyaloka and Satyamani Quartz, Scolecite, Sedona Stone, Shaman Quartz, Stellar Beam Calcite, Trigonic Quartz, Violane, Z-stone. *Chakra:* soma, mid-hairline

   balance and align: Bytownite, Diaspore, Stellar Beam Calcite, Violane

   spin too rapid/stuck open: Isis Calcite, Pinky-beige Ussingite, Sedona Stone, Shaman Quartz, White Banded Agate

   spin too sluggish/stuck closed: Banded Agate, Diaspore, Nuummite, Preseli Bluestone

Sorcery: Nuummite, Purpurite

Soul: Anandalite, Brandenberg Amethyst, Cathedral Quartz, Golden Danburite, Nirvana Quartz, Trigonic Quartz. *Chakra:* higher crown, heart

Soul cleanser: Anandalite, Black Kyanite, Brandenberg Amethyst, Chinese Chromium Quartz, Chrysotile in Serpentine, Golden Danburite, Golden Healer, Khutnohorite, Prehnite with Epidote, Rutile with Hematite, Selenite, Smoky Cathedral Quartz, Smoky Elestial Quartz

Soul contracts, recognition and release: Agate, Banded Agate, Black Kyanite, Boli Stone, Botswana Agate, Brandenberg Amethyst, Charoite, Dumortierite, Flint, Gabbro, Green Aventurine, Kakortokite, Leopardskin Jasper, Pyrophyllite, Rainbow Mayanite, Red Amethyst, Wind Fossil Agate, Wulfenite. *Chakra:* past life, higher crown, causal vortex

Soul, dark night of: Celtic Quartz, Golden Danburite, Khutnohorite, Stone of Sanctuary, Tanzine Aura Quartz

Soul encrustations: Ethiopian Opal

Soul evolution: Hilulite, Paraiba Tourmaline, Shift Crystal

Soul fragmentation: Anandalite, Angel's Wing Calcite, Brandenberg, Selenite. *Chakra*: past life

Soul growth: Agrellite, Beryllonite, Epidote

Soul healing: Amphibole, Anandalite, Black Kyanite, Blue Aragonite, Brandenberg Amethyst, Cassiterite, Ethiopian Opal, Fiskenaesset Ruby, Golden Healer, Khutnohorite, Marble, Nuummite, Pink Lazurine, Porphyrite (Chinese Letter Stone), Preseli Bluestone, Ruby Lavender Quartz, Trigonic Quartz

Soul imperatives: Nirvana Quartz, Porphyrite (Chinese Letter Stone), Tantalite

Soul, incarnate fully: Bushman Red Cascade Quartz, Celestial Quartz, Snakeskin Agate

Soul memory: Amphibole, Anandalite, Ancestralite, Brandenberg Amethyst, Cacoxenite, Cradle of Life (Humankind), Datolite, Trigonic Quartz

Soul, overcome fear: Amphibole, Golden Healer,

Khutnohorite, Stone of Sanctuary, Revelation Stone, Tangerose

Soul overlay: Brandenberg Amethyst, Scheelite

Soul path/plan: Amblygonite, Anthrophyllite, Astrophyllite, Black Kyanite, Blue Aragonite, Brazilianite, Candle Quartz, Cathedral Quartz, Crystalline Kyanite, Datolite, Golden Danburite, Icicle Calcite, Indicolite Quartz, Khutnohorite, Lemurian Jade, Leopardskin Serpentine, Lepidocrocite, Merkabite Calcite, Paraiba Tourmaline, Rainbow Mayanite, Rainbow Moonstone, Stellar Beam Calcite

Soul parts/spirits in the shamanic middle world: Celestobarite, Selenite

Soul parts, storage after retrieval: Brandenberg Amethyst, Clear Kunzite, Fulgarite, Selenite

Soul retrieval: Epidote, Faden Quartz, Flint, Fulgarite, Gaspeite, Khutnohorite, Mount Shasta Opal, Nuummite, Preseli Bluestone, Rainbow Mayanite, Snakeskin Agate, Tangerose. *Chakra:* higher heart, third eye

Soul star chakra: Afghanite, Ajoite, Amethyst Elestial, Amphibole, Anandalite, Angel's Wing Calcite, Apophyllite, Astraline, Auralite 23, Azeztulite, Blue Flint, Brandenberg Amethyst, Celestite, Celestobarite, Chevron Amethyst, Citrine, Danburite, Dianite, Diaspore (Zultanite), Elestial Quartz, Fire and Ice, Fire and Ice and Nirvana Quartz, Golden Enhydro Herkimer, Golden Himalayan Azeztulite, Green Ridge Quartz, Hematite, Herkimer Diamond, Holly Agate, Keyiapo, Khutnohorite, Kunzite, Lapis Lazuli, Lavender Quartz,

Merkabite Calcite, Muscovite, Natrolite, Novaculite, Nuummite, Onyx, Orange River Quartz, Petalite, Phenacite, Phenacite in Feldspar, Prophecy Stone, Purple Siberian Quartz, Purpurite, Quartz, Rainbow Mayanite, Rosophia, Satyamani and Satyaloka Quartz, Scolecite, Selenite, Shungite, Snowflake Obsidian, Spirit Quartz, Stellar Beam Calcite, Sugilite, Tangerine Aura Quartz, Tanzanite, Tanzine Aura Quartz, Titanite (Sphene), Trigonic Quartz, Vera Cruz Amethyst, Violane, White Elestial. *Chakra:* soul star, a foot or so above head

> **balance and align:** Anandalite, Vera Cruz Amethyst, Violane
>
> **spin too rapid/stuck open:** Celestobarite, Novaculite, Nuummite, Pinky-beige Ussingite, White, Rose or Smoky Elestial Quartz
>
> **spin too sluggish/stuck closed:** Golden Himalayan Azeztulite, Petalite, Phenacite, Rosophia

Speech impediments: Black Moonstone, Blue Crackle Quartz, Blue Euclase, Blue Lace Agate, Sodalite, Spider Web Obsidian, Sugilite. *Chakra:* third eye, throat

Spirit attachment: Aegerine, Avalonite, Blue Selenite, Brandenberg Amethyst, Brown Jasper, Celestobarite, Chlorite Quartz, Citrine Herkimer, Datolite, Drusy Golden Healer, Flint, Fluorite, Halite, Herkimer Diamond, Iolite, Klinopotilolith, Kunzite, Labradorite, Larimar, Larvikite, Laser Quartz, Lemurian Seed, Libyan Gold Tektite, Marcasite, Nirvana Quartz, Petalite, Phantom Selenite, Pyrolusite, Pyromorphite, Rainbow Mayanite, Selenite Wand, Shattuckite, Smoky Amethyst,

Smoky Citrine, Smoky Elestial, Smoky Phantom Quartz, Spirit Quartz, Stibnite, Tektite, Yellow Phantom Quartz. *Chakra:* soma chakra, solar plexus, third eye or heart

ascertain where or what attachment is: Aegerine, Apophyllite, Blue (Indicolite) Tourmaline, Celestobarite, Chrysolite, Quartz with Mica. *Chakra:* third eye

release disembodied spirits attached to places: Larimar, Marcasite, Smoky Amethyst. Leave in the room or site (the effect is enhanced if you add Petaltone Astral Clear or Z14 essence).

release mental attachments: Aegerine, Blue Halite, Limonite, Pyrolusite, Smoky Amethyst, Yellow Phantom Quartz. *Chakra:* third eye, soma, causal vortex

releasing attachment: Aegerine, Amethyst, Avalonite, Blue Selenite, Brandenberg Amethyst, Brown Jasper, Celestobarite, Citrine Herkimer, Datolite, Fluorite, Halite, Herkimer Diamond, Iolite, Kunzite, Labradorite, Larimar, Laser Quartz, Marcasite, Petalite, Phantom Quartz, Pyrolusite, Selenite Wand, Shattuckite, Smoky Citrine, Smoky Elestial, Smoky Quartz, Spirit Quartz, Stibnite, Yellow Phantom Quartz. *Chakra:* soma, solar plexus or heart

remove ancestral attachment: Ancestralite, Brandenberg Amethyst, Cradle of Life (Humankind), Datolite (attachment carried in the genes), Fairy Quartz, Lakelandite, Petrified Wood, Rainforest Jasper, Smoky Elestial, Spirit Quartz. *Chakra:* soma chakra or solar plexus

remove disembodied spirits after channelling or other metaphysical activity: Banded Agate, Botswana Agate, Shattuckite. *Chakra:* third eye

remove 'implants': Dravide (Brown) Tourmaline, Flint, Purple Tourmaline, Rainbow Mayanite, Smoky Amethyst. Place over site.

repair aura after removal: Aegerine, Anandalite, Celtic Quartz, Faden Quartz, Laser Quartz, Phantom Quartzes, Quartz, Selenite, Stibnite

Spirit release: Chlorite Quartz, Flint, Jasper Knife, Nirvana Quartz, Nuummite, Obsidian, Rainbow Mayanite, Spirit Quartz, Stibnite. *Chakra:* as appropriate

Spirits attached to places: Celtic Quartz, Larimar, Marcasite, Smoky Amethyst, Smoky Quartz

Spirits attached to third eye: Anandalite, Brandenberg Amethyst, Celestobarite, Larimar, Laser Quartz, Petalite, Petoskey Stone, Pyrolusite, Shattuckite, Smoky Amethyst, Smoky Phantom Quartz. *Chakra:* third eye

Spirits, release from chakras: Flint, Lemurian Seed, Petalite, Rainbow Mayanite, Smoky Amethyst, and see chakra entries

Spleen chakra: Amber, Aventurine, Bloodstone, Carnelian, Chlorite Quartz, Emerald, Eye of the Storm, Fire Opal, Flint, Gaspeite, Green Aventurine, Green Fluorite, Jade, Orange River Quartz, Prasiolite, Rhodochrosite, Rhodonite, Ruby, Tugtupite, Zircon. *Chakra:* under left armpit

balance and align: Charoite, Emerald, Eye of the

Storm, Flint, Green Aventurine, Tugtupite

clear attachments and hooks: Aventurine, Chert, Flint, Gaspeite, Jade, Jasper, Lemurian Seed

right armpit: Bloodstone, Eye of the Storm, Gaspeite, Triplite, Tugtupite

spin too rapid/stuck open: Amber, Aventurine, Chlorite Quartz, Eye of the Storm, Flint, Gaspeite, Green Fluorite, Jade, Prasiolite, Tugtupite

spin too sluggish/stuck closed: Fire Opal, Orange River Quartz, Rhodonite, Ruby, Topaz

Stagnant energy: Chlorite Quartz, Chrome Diopside, Citrine, Eye of the Storm, Garnet in Quartz, Golden Healer, Pinolith, Poppy Jasper, Quartz, Ruby Lavender Quartz, Sedona Stone, Selenite, Shaman Quartz, Smoky Elestial Quartz, Smoky Quartz, Tantalite, Triplite, and see Negative energy page 345. *Chakra:* base, dantien

Star children: Calcite Fairy Stone, Empowerite, Fairy Quartz, Glaucophane, Star Hollandite, Starseed Quartz. *Chakra:* higher crown

State stones: see Country and state stones page 304

Stellar gateway chakra: Afghanite, Ajoite, Amethyst Elestial, Amphibole, Anandalite™, Angelinite, Angel's Wing Calcite, Apophyllite, Astraline, Azeztulite, Brandenberg Amethyst, Celestite, Dianite, Diaspore (Zultanite), Elestial Quartz, Fire and Ice, Golden Himalayan Azeztulite, Golden Selenite, Green Ridge Quartz, Holly Agate, Ice Quartz, Kunzite, Merkabite Calcite, Moldavite, Nirvana Quartz, Novaculite, Petalite, Phenacite, Purpurite, Stellar Beam Calcite, Titanite

(Sphene), Trigonic Quartz, White Elestial Quartz. *Chakra:* arm's length above head

> **balance and align:** Ajoite, Amethyst Elestial, Anandalite, Brandenberg Amethyst, Kunzite
>
> **spin too rapid/stuck open:** Amphibole Quartz, Ice Quartz, Merkabite Calcite, Pinky-beige Ussingite, Purpurite
>
> **spin too sluggish/stuck closed:** Angel's Wing Calcite, Blue Celtic Quartz, Diaspore, Phenacite

Stuck souls and inappropriate 'crystal mentors': Aegerine, Anandalite, Banded Agate, Botswana Agate, Candle Quartz, Flint, Jet, Quartz, Rainbow Mayanite, Rose Quartz, Shattuckite, Smoky Amethyst, Smoky or Amethyst Brandenberg, Spirit Quartz, Stibnite, Super 7. *Chakra:* soma, third eye, causal vortex or place in environment

Subconscious blocks: Lepidocrocite, Molybdenite in Quartz, Smoky Elestial Quartz, Smoky Spirit Quartz. *Chakra:* dantien, soul star, stellar gateway, causal vortex, third eye, soma

Subtle energy bodies:

> **ancestral:** Ancestralite, Anthrophyllite, Blue Holly Agate, Brandenberg Amethyst, Bumble Bee Jasper, Candle Quartz, Catlinite, Cradle of Life (Humankind), Datolite, Eclipse Stone, Fairy Quartz, Golden Healer, Icicle Calcite, Ilmenite, Jade, Kambaba Jasper, Lakelandite, Lemurian Aquitane Calcite, Mohawkite, Peanut Wood, Petrified Wood, Porphyrite, Prasiolite, Rainbow Mayanite, Rainforest Jasper, Shaman Quartz,

Smoky Elestial Quartz, Spirit Quartz, Starseed, Stromatolite. *Chakra:* soul star, past life, alta major, causal vortex, higher heart, earth star and Gaia gateway

emotional: Apache Tear, Black Moonstone, Blue Moonstone, Botswana (Banded) Agate, Brandenberg Amethyst, Calcite, Danburite, Golden Healer, Icicle Calcite, Kunzite, Lepidolite, Mangano Calcite, Moonstone, Pink Moonstone, Pink Petalite, Rainbow Mayanite, Rainbow Moonstone, Rainbow Obsidian, Rhodochrosite, Rhodonite, Rose Elestial Quartz, Rose Quartz, Rubellite, Selenite, Tourmalinated Quartz, Tugtupite, Watermelon Tourmaline. *Chakra:* solar plexus, three-chambered heart, sacral and base chakras, knees and feet

etheric: Andescine Labradorite, Angelinite, Astraline, Brandenberg Amethyst, Chlorite Quartz, Chrysotile, Cradle of Life (Humankind), Datolite, Elestial Quartz, Ethiopian Opal, Eye of the Storm, Flint, Girasol, Golden Healer, Icicle Calcite, Keyiapo, Khutnohorite, Lemurian Aquitane Calcite, Poldervaarite, Pollucite, Quantum Quattro, Que Sera, Rainbow Mayanite, Rhodozite, Ruby Lavender Quartz, Sanda Rosa Azeztulite, Scheelite, Selenite, Shaman Quartz, Shungite, Stellar Beam Calcite, Tangerine Dream Lemurian, Tantalite. *Chakra:* 7 traditional chakras, plus soma, past life, alta major, causal vortex

karmic/karmic blueprint: Ammolite, Ammonite, Ancestralite, Brandenberg Amethyst, Cloudy Quartz,

Cradle of Life (Humankind), Crinoidal Limestone, Datolite, Dumortierite, Flint, Kambaba Jasper, Keyiapo, Khutnohorite, Lemurian Seed, Nirvana Quartz, Rainbow Mayanite, Rhodozite, Ruby Lavender Quartz, Sanda Rosa Azeztulite, Scheelite, Shaman Quartz, Shungite, Stromatolite, Titanite (Sphene), and see page 336. *Chakra:* past life, alta major, causal vortex, soma, knee and earth star

lightbody: Agnitite™, Amazez, Anandalite™, Angel's Wing Calcite, Azeztulite, Blue Moonstone, Brandenberg Amethyst, Chlorite Brandenberg, Eklogite, Erythrite, Golden Coracalcite, Golden Healer Quartz, Golden Himalayan Azeztulite, Hackmanite, Himalayan Gold Azeztulite™, Lemurian Seed, Lilac-purple Coquimbite, Madagascan Red Celestial Quartz, Mahogany Sheen Obsidian, Merkabite Calcite, Natrolite, Nirvana Quartz, Opal Aura Quartz, Phantom Calcite, Phenacite, Pink Lemurian, Prophecy Stone, Rainbow Mayanite, Red Amethyst, Rutilated Quartz (Angel Hair), Rutile with Hematite, Satyaloka Quartz, Satyamani Quartz, Scolecite, Spirit Quartz, Sugar Blade Quartz, Tangerine Dream Lemurian, Tiffany Stone, Trigonic Quartz, Tugtupite, Vera Cruz Amethyst, Violet Ussingite. *Chakra:* soma, soul star, stellar gateway, Gaia gateway, alta major, causal vortex

mental: Amechlorite, Amethyst, Arfvedsonite, Auralite 23, Brandenberg Amethyst, Celadonite, Chlorite Brandenberg, Crystal Cap Amethyst,

Dumortierite, Fluorite, Lemurian Seed, Merkabite Calcite, Nuummite, Owyhee Blue Opal, Rainbow Covellite, Rainbow Mayanite, Sapphire, Scheelite, Scolecite, Sodalite, Sugilite, Vera Cruz Amethyst. *Chakra:* third eye, soma, alta major, causal vortex

physical, subtle: Amechlorite, Anandalite, Ancestralite, Bloodstone, Brandenberg Amethyst, Carnelian, Cradle of Life (Humankind), Dumortierite, Eilat Stone, Eklogite, Flint, Hematite, Kambaba Jasper, Madagascan Red Celestial Quartz, Quantum Quattro, Que Sera, Rainbow Mayanite, Red Amethyst, Stromatolite. *Chakras:* base, sacral, dantien, earth star

planetary: Aswan Granite, Brandenberg Amethyst, Celtic Quartz, Charoite, Lapis Lazuli, Libyan Gold Tektite, Moldavite, Nebula Stone, Preseli Bluestone, Rainbow Mayanite, Starseed Quartz, Tektite, Trigonic. *Chakra:* past life, alta major, causal vortex, soma, stellar and Gaia gateway chakras

spiritual: Anandalite, Azeztulite, Brandenberg Amethyst, Golden Herkimer Diamond, Golden Quartz, Green Ridge Quartz, Larimar, Lemurian Seed, Nirvana Quartz, Phenacite, Rainbow Mayanite, Shaman Quartz, Trigonic Amethyst, Trigonic Quartz. *Chakra:* past life, soul star, stellar gateway, alta major, causal vortex

Survival instincts: Ammolite, Kimberlite, Thunder Egg. *Chakra:* base

Taking on other people's feelings or conditions: Black Tourmaline, Brochantite, Healer's Gold, Iridescent Pyrite, Labradorite, Lemurian Jade, Mohawkite. *Chakra:* solar plexus, spleen

Third eye (brow) chakra: Afghanite, Ajo Quartz, Ajoite, Amber, Amechlorite, Amethyst, Ammolite, Amphibole Quartz, Angelite, Apophyllite, Aquamarine, Axinite, Azurite, Black Moonstone, Blue Calcite, Blue Kyanite, Blue Lace Agate, Blue Obsidian, Blue Selenite, Blue Topaz, Blue Tourmaline, Bytownite (Yellow Labradorite), Cacoxenite, Cavansite, Champagne Aura Quartz, Diaspore, Electric-blue Obsidian, Eye of the Storm, Garnet, Glaucophane, Golden Himalayan Azeztulite, Herderite, Herkimer Diamond, Holly Agate, Howlite, Indigo Auram, Iolite, Kunzite, Labradorite, Lapis Lazuli, Lavender-purple Opal, Lazulite, Lepidolite, Libyan Gold Tektite, Malachite with Azurite (use as polished stone, make essence by indirect method), Moldavite, Petoskey Stone, Pietersite, Preseli Bluestone, Purple Fluorite, Rhomboid Selenite, Sapphire, Serpentine in Obsidian, Sodalite, Spectrolite, Stilbite, Sugilite, Tangerine Aura Quartz, Turquoise, Unakite, Yellow Labradorite (Bytownite). *Chakra:* above and between eyebrows

> **balance and align:** Anandalite, Black Moonstone, Sugilite
>
> **spin too rapid/stuck open:** Diaspore, Iolite, Lavender-purple Opal, Pietersite, Serpentine in Obsidian,

Sodalite, Sugilite

spin too sluggish/stuck closed: Apophyllite, Azurite, Banded Agate, Diaspore, Herkimer Diamond, Optical Calcite, Rhomboid Calcite, Rhomboid Selenite, Royal Blue Sapphire, Tanzine Aura Quartz, Yellow Labradorite (Bytownite)

Thought form, disperse: Aegerine, Blue Selenite, Brown Jasper, Celestobarite, Citrine Herkimer, Firework Obsidian, Herkimer Diamond, Iolite, Kunzite, Labradorite, Nuummite, Petoskey Stone, Pyrolusite, Rainbow Mayanite, Scolecite, Smoky Amethyst, Smoky Citrine, Spectrolite, Stibnite

Three-chambered heart chakra: Anandalite, Azeztulite, Danburite, Eudialyte, Petalite, Rhodozaz, Rose Elestial Quartz, Trigonic Quartz, Tugtupite

Throat chakra: Ajo Quartz, Ajoite, Amber, Amethyst, Aquamarine, Astraline, Azurite, Blue Chalcedony, Blue Kyanite, Blue Lace Agate, Blue Obsidian, Blue Quartz, Blue Topaz, Blue Tourmaline, Chalcanthite, Chrysocolla, Chrysotile, Eye of the Storm, Glaucophane, Green Ridge Quartz, Indicolite Quartz, Kunzite, Lapis Lazuli, Lepidolite, Moldavite, Paraiba Tourmaline, Sugilite, Turquoise. Place over throat.

balance and align: Anandalite, Blue Chalcedony, Blue Lace Agate, Blue Topaz, Indicolite Quartz, Sapphire

spin too rapid/stuck open: Black Sapphire, Lepidolite, Paraiba Tourmaline, Sugilite, Turquoise

spin too sluggish/stuck closed: Chrysocolla, Lapis Lazuli, Moldavite, Turquoise

Throat issues: Astraline, Blue Lace Agate, Blue Quartz, Chalcanthite, Glaucophane, Green Ridge Quartz, Indicolite Quartz, Paraiba Tourmaline (place over throat)

Tics: Fenster Quartz, and see twitches page 383

Tie cutting: Flint, Green Aventurine, Green Obsidian, Jasper Knife, Laser Quartz, Leopardskin Jasper, Malachite (use as polished stone, make remedy by indirect method), Novaculite, Petalite, Rainbow Mayanite, Rainbow Obsidian, Stibnite, Sunstone, Wulfenite. *Chakra:* past life, base, sacral, solar plexus, brow

Timelines: Ancestralite, Brandenberg Amethyst, Chrysotile, Cradle of Life (Humankind), Dumortierite, Shiva Shell. *Chakra:* past life, causal vortex

Tinnitus: Alabandite, Ammolite, Dogtooth Calcite, Ocean Jasper, Peanut Wood, Serpentine, Xenotine. Use over ear or on past life chakra.

Trauma: Amethyst, Ammolite, Blue Euclase, Bornite, Brandenberg Amethyst, Cathedral Quartz, Cavansite, Dumortierite, Empowerite, Epidote, Eye of the Storm, Faden Quartz, Fulgarite, Gaia Stone, Garnet in Quartz, Green Diopside, Green Ridge Quartz, Goethite, Golden Healer, Guardian Stone, Kimberlite, Mangano Vesuvianite, Novaculite with Nuummite, Ocean Blue Jasper, Oregon Opal, Peach Selenite, Peanut Wood, Prasiolite, Richterite, Ruby Lavender Quartz, Scapolite, Sea Sediment Jasper, Smoky Elestial, Spirit Quartz, Tantalite, Victorite, Wavellite, Youngite. *Chakra:* solar plexus, or wear constantly

Trust: Rhodolite Garnet

Truth, speak: Astraline, Blue Lace Agate, Morganite with Azeztulite. *Chakra:* throat

Tummy button: see Navel page 345

Twitches/tics: Amethyst, Apache Tear, Azurite, Blue Aragonite, Cerussite, Chrysocolla, Magnesite, Magnetite (Lodestone), Rose Quartz. Place over site.

– U –

Unacceptable thoughts and feelings: Amazez, Anandalite, Auralite 23, Golden Healer, Scolecite, Vivianite. *Chakra:* solar plexus, third eye

Unconditional love: Astraline, Cobalto Calcite, Erythrite, Luvulite, Rose Quartz, Sugilite, Tangerose, Tugtupite. *Chakra:* higher heart (wear continuously or place over higher heart)

Unconditional self-love: Citrine, Emerald, Erythrite, Luvulite, Mangano Calcite, Pink Calcite, Rose Quartz, Sugilite, Tugtupite

Uncursing: Black Tourmaline, Novaculite, Nuummite, Purpurite, Stibnite, Tourmalinated Quartz

Undue mental influence/attachments: Aegerine, Blue Halite, Limonite, Pyrolusite, Smoky Amethyst, Yellow Phantom Quartz

Ungroundedness: Aztee, Basalt, Boji Stone, Celestobarite, Chlorite Quartz, Dragon Stone, Empowerite, Flint, Granite, Graphic Smoky Quartz (Zebra Stone), Hematite, Kambaba Jasper, Mohawkite, Peanut Wood, Polychrome Jasper, Proustite, Serpentine in Obsidian, Shell Jasper, Smoky Elestial Quartz, Steatite, Stromatolite. *Chakra:* earth star, base, dantien, Gaia gateway. Or place behind knees.

Unification and integration crystals: Anandalite, Aura Quartz, Auralite 23, Brandenberg Amethyst, Included Quartz, K2, Lapis Lazuli, Lavender Aragonite, Lodolite, Menalite, Moldavite, Pink Granite, Polychrome Jasper,

Preseli Bluestone, Quantum Quattro, Selenite, Shiva Lingam, Spirit Quartz, Tektite, Turquoise. *Chakra:* dantien

– V –

Vacillation: Brucite, Shiva Lingam. *Chakra:* dantien

Vampirism of heart energy: Aventurine, Gaspeite, Greenlandite, Iridescent Pyrite, Lemurian Aquitane Calcite, Mangano Calcite, Nunderite, Tantalite, Xenotine. *Chakra:* solar plexus, heart, higher heart

Vampirism of spleen energy: Gaspeite, Green Aventurine, Green Fluorite, Iridescent Pyrite, Jade, Nunderite, Tantalite, Xenotine. *Chakra:* spleen

Vibrational change, facilitate: Anandalite, Bismuth, Celtic Healer Quartz, Gabbro, Huebnerite, Lemurian Gold Opal, Lemurian Jade, Luxullianite, Montebrasite, Mtrolite, Nunderite, Rainbow Mayanite, Rosophia, Sanda Rosa Azeztulite, Snakeskin Pyrite, Sonora Sunrise, Trigonic Quartz. *Chakra:* higher heart, higher crown. Wear stones frequently or keep within reach and hold frequently.

Victim mentality: Amblygonite, Brazilianite, Epidote, Green Ridge Quartz, Hematoid Calcite, Ice Quartz, Marcasite, Orange River Quartz, Rose Quartz, Smoky Lemurian Seed, Tugtupite with Nuummite, Zircon. *Chakra:* dantien

Violence, negate: Eye of the Storm (Judy's Jasper). *Chakra:* base (keep in environment)

Visualisation: Annabergite, Apophyllite pyramid, Azurite, Blue or Rhomboid Calcite, Golden Labradorite (Bytownite), Lapis Lazuli, Prehnite, Selenite or Blue Selenite. *Chakra:* third eye

Vocal cords: Blue Aragonite, Blue Lace Agate, Hackmanite, Indicolite Quartz, Lemurian Aquitane Calcite, Owyhee Blue Opal. *Chakra:* throat, wear or take as crystal essence

– W –

War-gene, dissolve: Anandalite, Ancestralite, Brandenberg Amethyst, Rose Quartz, Trigonic Quartz. *Chakra:* causal vortex, base and sacral

Wisdom: Amphibole Quartz, Anandalite, Atlantasite, Avalonite, Bytownite, Calligraphy Stone, Cathedral Quartz, Chrysotile, Covellite, Creedite, Dumortierite, Eilat Stone, Golden Danburite, Golden Herkimer, Greenlandite, Hanksite, Lemurian Seed, Leopardskin Jasper, Libyan Gold Tektite, Merlinite, Nirvana Quartz, Ocean Jasper, Ouro Verde, Paraiba Tourmaline, Peach Selenite, Sichuan Quartz, Spectrolite, Star Hollandite, Starseed Quartz, Stellar Beam Calcite, Tibetan Black Spot Quartz, Trigonic Quartz, Ussingite. *Chakra:* crown

Worry, excessive: Pink Crackle Quartz, Revelation Stone, Snakeskin Agate, Sonora Sunrise

Wounds, imprints in etheric body: Ajoite, Ancestralite, Andean Blue Opal, Atlantasite, Bixbite, Cradle of Life (Humankind), Diaspore (Zultanite), Flint, Gaia Stone, Golden Healer, Klinoptilolith, Lakelandite, Mookaite Jasper, Pumice, Quantum Quattro, Sceptre Quartz, Schalenblende, Seriphos Quartz, Shungite, Smoky Amethyst, Tibetan Black Spot Quartz, Youngite. *Chakra:* past life or over site

– X –

Xiphoid process: see Heart seed chakra

– Y –

Yin-yang imbalances: Alunite, Amphibole Quartz, Dalmatian Stone, Day and Night Quartz, Eilat Stone, Morion, Poppy Jasper, Scheelite, Shiva Lingam, Spirit Quartz. *Chakra:* base, dantien

– Z –

Zealot: Amblygonite, Smoky Quartz
Ziggurat: Bloodstone, Carnelian, Selenite
Zoroastrianism: Fire Agate, Fire Obsidian
Zygote damaged: Ancestralite, Brandenberg Amethyst, Celtic Chevron Quartz, Cradle of Life (Humankind), Menalite

Footnotes

1. http://www.ufodigest.com/news/0706/dnamemory.html

2. http://www.tantrikstudies.org/blog/2016/3/3/why-spiritual-growth-does-not-lead-to-enlightenment

3. Original copyright holder unascertainable.

4. *The new data come from the Encyclopedia of DNA Elements project, or ENCODE, a $123 million endeavour begun by the National Human Genome Research Institute (NHGRI) in 2003, which includes 442 scientists in 32 labs around the world.* http://healthland.time.com/2012/09/06/junk-dna-not-so-useless-after-all/

5. https://www.reddit.com/r/evolution/comments/3d30ip/is_junk_dna_simply_ancestral_dna_that_we_no/

6. "Pseudogenes", *Comparative and Functional Genomics*. 2012; 2012: 424526. NCBI, National Institutes of Health:

   http://www.ncbi.nlm.nih.gov/pmc/articles/PMC3352212/

7. Joseph R. Scogna, Jr., *Light, Dark: The Neuron and the Axon*

8. Joseph R. Scogna, Jr. and Kathy Scogna, *Junk DNA*

9. See for instance the work of Dr Valerie Hunt, *Infinite Mind* (no longer in print but available as an e-book from her website): http://www.valerievhunt.com/ValerieVHunt.com/Valerie_Hunt_EdD.html (consulted April 2014)

10. http://www.earthspectrum.com/healing/scalaren

ergy-system.htm (consulted April 2014)

11. "Crystals of the brain", *EMBO Molecular Medicine*. 2011 Feb; 3(2): 69–71.
    http://www.ncbi.nlm.nih.gov/pmc/articles/PMC3377059/

12. "Understanding how your mind can heal your brain."
    https://biacolorado.org/biac/wp-content/uploads/2013/07/Copy-of-Brainstorm-2.pdf

13. http://www.sciencedirect.com/science/article/pii/S0304416598001603

14. Kahane-Nissenbaum, Melissa C., "Exploring Intergenerational Transmission of Trauma in Third Generation Holocaust Survivors" (2011). *Doctorate in Social Work (DSW) Dissertations*. Paper 16:
    http://repository.upenn.edu/edissertations_sp2/16/

15. Discovermagazine.com/2013/may/13-grandmas-experiences-leave-epigenetic-mark-on-your-genes

16. 1 December 2013, "Fear of a smell can be passed down several generations", Linda Geddes:
    https://www.newscientist.com/article/dn24677-fear-of-a-smell-can-be-passed-down-several-generations/

17. http://www.sakino.de/the-healing-power-of-family-and-systemic-constellation-work/

Resources

Crystal suppliers

Crystals specially charged for you by Judy Hall are available at www.angeladditions.co.uk

USA: Excellent high vibration crystals are available from www.exquisitecrystals.com

and http://www.neatstuff.net/avalon

UK: www.hehishelo.co.uk and www.ksccrystals.com

Crystal cleansers

Clear2Light from www.petaltone.co.uk is an excellent crystal cleanser and is available worldwide via www.petaltoneusa.com. Crystal Charge is also available from Petaltone, as is Z14 which clears fourteen layers of the etheric.

Crystal Cleanser spray from the Crystal Balance Company and Crystal Recharge along with transmuting Violet Flame work wonders (www.crystalbalance.net).

Green Man Essences:
http://www.greenmanshop.co.uk/acatalog/Essences.html

Crystal essence for addiction

Addiction, Cravings and Dependency:
http://www.crystal-alchemy.com/addiction.php

Further reading by Judy Hall

Crystal Prescriptions 1–5 (O-Books, Arlesford, 2005)

Earth Blessings: Using Crystals for Personal Energy Clearing,

Earth Healing & Environmental Enhancement (Watkins Publishing, 2014)

The Book of Why (Flying Horse, 2010)

The Soulmate Myth (Flying Horse, 2010)

Patterns of the Past (The Wessex Astrologer, 2000)

Karmic Connections (The Wessex Astrologer, 2001)

The Crystal Wisdom Healing Oracle Kit (Watkins Books, London, 2016)(

Crystal Bibles, volumes 1–3 (Godsfield Press, London, UK; Walking Stick Press, USA)

Torn Clouds: a time slip novel (O-Books)

101 Power Crystals: The Ultimate Guide to Magical Crystals, Gems, and Stones for Healing and Transformation (Fair Winds, USA; Quarto, London)

Crystals and Sacred Sites: Use Crystals to Access the Power of Sacred Landscapes for Personal and Planetary Transformation (Fair Winds, USA, 2012)

The Crystal Experience: Your complete crystal workshop in a book (Godsfield, London, 2010)

The Encyclopedia of Crystals (Godsfield Press, UK; Fair Winds, USA, revised edition 2015)

Psychic Self-Protection: Using Crystals to Change Your Life (Hay House, 2009)

Good Vibrations: Psychic Protection, Energy Enhancement and Space Clearing (Flying Horse Publications, Bournemouth, 2008)

Life-Changing Crystals: Using crystals to manifest abundance, wellbeing and happiness (Godsfield Press, UK, 2013); *Crystals to Empower You* (F&W, USA, 2013)

20 Minutes to Master: Past Life Therapy: The Only Introduction You'll Ever Need, e-book (HarperCollins, UK, August 2013)

Other authors

Cunningham, Donna, and Andrew Ramer, *Spiritual Dimensions of Healing Addictions*

(Cassandra Press, 1 November 1988)

Cunningham, Donna, and Andrew Ramer, *Further Dimensions of Healing Addictions* (Cassandra Press, March 1989)

Kaehr, Shelley, *Past Lives with Gems & Stones* (CreateSpace Independent Publishing Platform, June 15, 2014)

Koch, Liz, *The Psoas Book: A Comprehensive Guide to the Iliopsoas Muscle and Its Effect on the Body/Mind/Emotions* (Guinea Pig Publications; PO Box 1226, Felton, CA 95018; www.guineapigpub.com)

Pearson, Nicholas, *Crystals for Karmic Healing* (Destiny Books, 2017)

Scogna, Joseph R., Jr. and Kathy M. Scogna, *Junk DNA: Unlocking the Hidden Secrets of Your DNA* (CreateSpace Independent Publishing Platform, September 27, 2014)

Internet resources

PTSD

A useful site that explores Post Traumatic Stress Disorder, how it arises and how it can be healed:

http://www.mind.org.uk/information-support/types-of-mental-health-problems/post-traumatic-stress-disorder-ptsd/useful-contacts/#.WIaMlbmTM34, http://www.ptsd uk.org/ (an online community for sufferers), https://www.helpguide.org/articles/ptsd-trauma/post-traumatic-stress-disorder.htm in the UK and Ireland, and https://medlineplus.gov/posttraumaticstressdisorder.ht ml in the US.

See http://healthland.time.com/2012/09/06/junk-dna-not-so-useless-after-all/ for an overview of 'junk DNA' and how it is presently viewed.

Transgenerational research

Kahane-Nissenbaum, Melissa C., "Exploring Intergenerational Transmission of Trauma in Third Generation Holocaust Survivors" (2011). *Doctorate in Social Work (DSW) Dissertations*. Paper 16.

Soul Retrieval research

There is very little evidential research available. These studies were completed under academic supervision:

"Shamanic Healing: A Qualitative Study Exploring the Effects of Soul Retrieval on Five Participants During One-to-Seven Years":

http://mariansimon.com/wp-content/uploads/2013/12/shamanic_healing-MarianSimon.pdf

"The Ancient Art of Shamanic Soul Retrieval":

www.creativespirit.net/learners/AUCulminatingProjects/cp-horst.pdf

Spirit Release/Soul Retrieval

Sandra Ingerman is probably the best known and most experienced teacher in the US and UK. See: http://www.sandraingerman.com/soulretrieval.html for a practitioner list.

Sue Allen is also a very experienced trainer who works in the UK and also South Africa: School of Intuition and Healing. See www.intuitionandhealing.co.uk for a practitioner list.

The UK Spirit Release Foundation has now closed its doors but they list trained therapists on:

http://www.spiritrelease.com/

Junk DNA, Kathy Scogna:

http://www.lifeenergyresearch.com/ and http://kathy-scogna.blogspot.co.uk/

BOOKS

O-BOOKS

SPIRITUALITY

O is a symbol of the world, of oneness and unity; this eye represents knowledge and insight. We publish titles on general spirituality and living a spiritual life. We aim to inform and help you on your own journey in this life. If you have enjoyed this book, why not tell other readers by posting a review on your preferred book site? Recent bestsellers from O-Books are:

Heart of Tantric Sex
Diana Richardson
Revealing Eastern secrets of deep love and intimacy to Western couples.
Paperback: 978-1-90381-637-0 ebook: 978-1-84694-637-0

Crystal Prescriptions
The A-Z guide to over 1,200 symptoms and their healing crystals
Judy Hall
The first in the popular series of six books, this handy little guide is packed as tight as a pill-bottle with crystal remedies for ailments.
Paperback: 978-1-90504-740-6 ebook: 978-1-84694-629-5

Take Me To Truth
Undoing the Ego
Nouk Sanchez, Tomas Vieira
The best-selling step-by-step book on shedding the Ego,
using the teachings of *A Course In Miracles*.
Paperback: 978-1-84694-050-7 ebook: 978-1-84694-654-7

The 7 Myths about Love...Actually!
The journey from your HEAD to the HEART
of your SOUL
Mike George
Smashes all the myths about LOVE.
Paperback: 978-1-84694-288-4 ebook: 978-1-84694-682-0

The Holy Spirit's Interpretation of the New Testament
A course in Understanding and Acceptance
Regina Dawn Akers
Following on from the strength of *A Course In Miracles*,
NTI teaches us how to experience the love and oneness
of God.
Paperback: 978-1-84694-085-9 ebook: 978-1-78099-083-5

The Message of A Course In Miracles
A translation of the text in plain language
Elizabeth A. Cronkhite
A translation of *A Course in Miracles* into plain, everyday
language for anyone seeking inner peace. The
companion volume, *Practicing A Course In Miracles*,
offers practical lessons and mentoring.

Paperback: 978-1-84694-319-5 ebook: 978-1-84694-642-4

Thinker's Guide to God
Peter Vardy
An introduction to key issues in the philosophy of
religion.
Paperback: 978-1-90381-622-6

Your Simple Path
Find happiness in every step
Ian Tucker
A guide to helping us reconnect with what is really
important in our lives.
Paperback: 978-1-78279-349-6 ebook: 978-1-78279-348-9

365 Days of Wisdom
Daily Messages To Inspire You Through The Year
Dadi Janki
Daily messages which cool the mind, warm the heart
and guide you along your journey.
Paperback: 978-1-84694-863-3 ebook: 978-1-84694-864-0

Body of Wisdom
Women's Spiritual Power and How it Serves
Hilary Hart
Bringing together the dreams and experiences of women
across the world with today's most visionary spiritual
teachers.
Paperback: 978-1-78099-696-7 ebook: 978-1-78099-695-0

Dying to Be Free
From Enforced Secrecy to Near Death to True
Transformation
Hannah Robinson
After an unexpected accident and near-death
experience, Hannah Robinson found herself radically
transforming her life, while a remarkable new insight
altered her relationship with her father; a practising
Catholic priest.
Paperback: 978-1-78535-254-6 ebook: 978-1-78535-255-3

**Readers of ebooks can buy or view any of these
bestsellers by clicking on the live link in the title.
Most titles are published in paperback and as an
ebook. Paperbacks are available in traditional
bookshops. Both print and ebook formats are
available online.**

**Find more titles and sign up to our readers'
newsletter at
http://www.johnhuntpublishing.com/mind-body-
spirit**

**Follow us on Facebook at
https://www.facebook.com/OBooks/
and Twitter at https://twitter.com/obooks**